Living with Arthritis

Everything You Need to Know

John Marcus Thompson, MD

FIREFLY BOOKS

A FIREFLY BOOK

Published by Firefly Books (U.S.) Inc. 2001

First Printing

U.S. CATALOGING-IN-PUBLICATION DATA
(Library of Congress Standards)

Thompson, John Marcus.
    Living with arthritis : everything you need to know / John Marcus Thompson. –1st ed.
[128] p. ; ill. :   cm. (Your personal health)
Includes index.
Summary: Understanding arthritis, its treatment, and ways to cope.
ISBN: 1-55209-611-4 (pbk)
1. Arthritis – Popular works. 2. Arthritis – Treatment – Popular works.
I. Title. II. Series.
616.7/22 21 2001   CIP

Published in the United States in 2001 by
Firefly Books (U.S.) Inc.
P.O. Box 1338, Ellicott Station
Buffalo, New York, USA
14205

Published in Canada in 2000 by Key Porter Books Limited.

Electronic formatting: Heidy Lawrance Associates
Diagrams: Martyn Lengden

Printed and bound in Canada

Contents

Acknowledgments

The professionals of the London office of the Arthritis Society, and in particular Nancy Ambrogio, Janet Goodhoofd, Joanne Cuttiford and Tammy Regier, have contributed significantly to this book, both as constructive critics and (in the section on therapy) as co-authors. They deserve my public thanks.

Several patients read individual sections and helped me with their comments. Of course, in a larger sense, my patients have made an enormous contribution over the years to my understanding of arthritis. My thanks, though, go beyond that. Few non-physicians can guess the rewards arising from what is rather cryptically called "the doctor-patient relationship." For trust, for understanding, for friendship, for all these I thank those I've been permitted to know and care for over the last quarter-century.

Finally, in countless ways Ana Thompson made this book possible.

Thank you all.

John M. Thompson, MD

Dedication

When I first met Carol, she was 24 years old. Her joint symptoms had begun four years earlier with the birth of her son, improved when she got pregnant again and returned for good when her daughter was born just a few months before that first visit.

Carol died 19 years later, almost to the day.

Over those years I got to know Carol well. We went through so much together: countless surgical procedures; virtually every drug then available; complications of arthritis that I had never seen before and have seldom seen since. Carol was in and out of hospital innumerable times, particularly in her final years. A crisis would force her to come in, and as soon as she was even partially better she would press to be discharged, to be home with her family. Finally, her life became impossible. She anticipated her death, and both she and Paul, her husband, were ready for it.

Carol had a mischievous, infectious sense of humor. She wasn't above taking gentle pokes at "the doctor," and I took these as a compliment. She shared a birthday with my wife, and every May 8 a card and a box of homemade cookies would be delivered to my office. The last few years, it was Paul or one of her children, now grown, who came by.

Carol dealt with her disease with grace and acceptance. Probably more than any other patient, she taught me about arthritis, about being a doctor, about living. This book is for her.

Author's Note

I've gone into detail in many sections of this book because I believe patients want and need detail. I feel strongly that in order to have the best possible outcome and avoid misadventure, patients must know as much about their arthritis as their doctor knows. This book is not simply an introduction; it is a manual, to be referred to repeatedly as circumstances change.

But because things do change – in particular with drug dosages and precautions – specifics should be checked with a health professional (a physician, pharmacist or nurse) if there is a discrepancy between what I have written and what the reader has been told.

Preface

Acommon aphorism states that knowledge is power. This principle certainly applies to consumers of medical care. Recent changes in health-care delivery require people to make more of their own decisions about how and where they will obtain care. Research findings clearly show that people who understand their illness and actively participate in treatment decisions have better outcomes and greater satisfaction.

The new emphasis on health-care costs and efficiency means that doctors often don't have adequate time to talk with their patients. Studies have consistently shown that the doctor's office is not a good setting for learning. Also, patients are often too upset, or too deferential to the doctor, to press for answers. Moreover, the doctor can't judge exactly what each patient needs to learn. Given these realities, patients must increasingly take responsibility for educating themselves.

This eminently readable book is a comprehensive resource for people with arthritis who wish to learn more about this very common group of illnesses. They should use it to make themselves more informed participants in the care of their illness, and to identify specific issues to discuss with their physicians. Most important, they should use it to help themselves feel more in charge of the illness, and of their lives.

Robert F. Meenan, MD, MPH, MBA
Director, Boston University School of Public Health

Anatomy of the skeleton

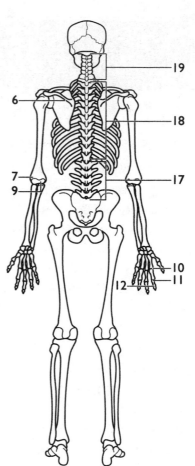

1 temporomandibular
   (TM or jaw) joint
2 sternoclavicular joint
3 sternum (breast bone)
4 clavicle (collar bone)
5 acromioclavicular joint
6 scapula (shoulder blade)
7 lateral epicondyle

8 medial epicondyle
9 elbow
10 metacarpophalangeal
   (MCP) joint
11 proximal interphalangeal
   (PIP) joint
12 distal interphalangeal
   (DIP) joint

13 greater trochanter
14 patella (knee cap)
15 metatarsophalangeal
   (MTP) joint
16 sacroiliac joint
17 lumbar spine
18 dorsal (thoracic) spine
19 cervical spine

ONE

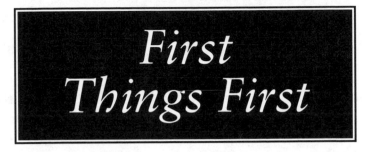

First
Things First

Rheumatology is the name given to the medical specialty that deals with people who have problems with their joints. Diagnosis and non-surgical treatment of these is the focus. Since a joint problem is often not the only one the patient has, the specialty spills over to include diseases that also affect muscles, the nerves, the blood, the skin, the kidneys, in fact, almost every part of the body.

I am a rheumatologist. After medical school I went on to spend three years learning the art of general internal medicine, and a further two years working exclusively with people with arthritis. For a little over 30 years I have been a practicing rheumatologist. Several days each week, I see patients who are referred to me because of joint pain.

Very often, after I've completed my examination, my patient will ask, "Tell me, doctor, is it arthritis?" The diagnosis may be one of a dozen very different conditions – osteoarthritis of the big toe, rheumatoid arthritis, back pain and gout are all common – but my answer to that particular question has to be "Yes." I then have to go on to explain, because I know that my patient is thinking, "Wheelchair."

I explain that "arthritis" means, literally, "joint inflammation." I add that we, doctors and patients, have come to lump just about anything that hurts in the muscles and the skeleton under this heading. My grandparents would have used the term "rheumatism."

"Arthritis" includes dozens of different conditions. Some are temporary, some are permanent. Some are harmless and some are disabling. Some are curable, some are not. So the word "arthritis," as most of us use it, is meaningless. We must be specific. That's the purpose of this book – to be specific, and to give meaning to the specific.

Another term to describe what we often call "arthritis" or "rheumatism" is "musculoskeletal disorder" (MSD). MSDs include joint disease (about 60 percent), back and neck pain (about 30 percent) and a wide variety of other problems, including tendinitis and bursitis (about 10 percent).

The 1990 Ontario Health Survey helps to put MSDs in perspective. This survey, which roughly confirms what earlier studies in Canada and the United States had shown, pointed out that roughly 14 percent of all adults are affected by MSDs (or between 3 and 4 million Canadians). This is equivalent to the entire population of British Columbia.

Estimates of some of the more common types of adult MSDs:

• osteoarthritis	1 in 10
• fibromyalgia	4 in 100
• rheumatoid arthritis	1 in 100
• crystal arthritis	1 in 100
• ankylosing spondylitis	1 in 1,000
• psoriatic arthritis	1 in 1,000
• systemic lupus	1 in 2,000

MSDs cause long-term disability in one North American out of 20. This is more than twice the rate of disability from heart and lung disease *combined*. MSDs rank higher than heart and lung disorders as a reason for visiting the doctor, and rank just after coughs, colds and flu as a cause of "sick days." They are the second most common reason prescriptions are written (after high blood pressure) or over-the-counter pills are purchased (after colds and flu).

How to Use This Book

This book covers a lot of territory. Chapters 2, 3, 4 and 5 deal with specific types of arthritis, and for most readers just one or two will be of uppermost concern.

There are sections, however, that are generally relevant. The next section, "How a Diagnosis Is Made," is a good starting point for anyone, particularly someone who has just recently begun to hurt. The distinction between "inflammatory" and "non-inflammatory" pain is important.

Chapter 6, "What's Going On?," provides information on symptoms as they crop up in various parts of the body. Some may be part of a larger arthritic problem, but many are not. Some aren't important at all, except as a source of worry. This is a "how-to-do-it" chapter.

Finally, Chapter 7, "The Treatment of Arthritis," is very important and generally applicable. Almost every person with pain is treated with pills. Because these may harm as well as help, patients have to learn to recognize side effects as they arise. This chapter should help with that. It also touches on a number of treatment possibilities that may not have been considered.

Obviously, this book is not meant to be read at a single sitting, but to be consulted, and reconsulted, over time.

How a Diagnosis Is Made

Ask any medical student how a diagnosis is made, and she or

he will answer, "Through a complete history, a thorough physical examination and appropriate laboratory tests."

This response, embedded in the medical profession's collective memory, was recently tested. Researchers in Texas presented a series of arthritis "cases" to a number of doctors. The problem cases were typical of those seen in practice – osteoarthritis, rheumatoid arthritis, back pain, gout, tendinitis and fibromyalgia were some of them. The doctors were all involved in general internal medicine, some were training to become specialists, and others were their teachers. This was a "paper" exercise; they didn't see the patients, but details of the history and physical examination were provided. They were asked to diagnose each case. To help them, they could order any test they felt was needed. Their performances were compared to the performances of a group of rheumatologists.

The outcome of the exercise was predictable. The doctors-in-training didn't do as well as their teachers, who in turn didn't do as well as the rheumatologists. Experience did count for something. Doctors who had been specialists for at least six years got 80 percent of the correct answers (the others were around 70 percent). It also helped if doctors had received some exposure to patients with arthritis. Two weeks on a rheumatology service made a big difference.

One fascinating part of the study has real relevance in today's cost-conscious world: to reach their incorrect diagnoses (three out of ten), the non-rheumatologists far outspent the arthritis doctors on unnecessary tests.

A fourth part should be added: "and a doctor with relevant experience." In other words, the cheapest and best "test" is a referral to an appropriate specialist. This is particularly important in rheumatology because – despite the fact that "rheumatism" makes up the largest part of general practice

– most of today's medical graduates have little or no experience with arthritis.

From the first moment I meet a new patient, I begin to collect information that will help answer two very important questions: "Is the problem inflammatory or non-inflammatory?" and "Is the problem local or widespread?"

Inflammatory or Non-inflammatory?

The answer to this question is very important. Generally, inflammatory arthritis:

- affects more joints
- causes more damage and disability
- is linked more often to problems elsewhere in the body
- is more likely to be influenced by treatment

Inflammation, whether due to sunburn, a mosquito bite or inflammatory arthritis, has four features: pain, swelling, redness and warmth. Rheumatoid arthritis, systemic lupus erythematosus (SLE) and gout are quite different but they all share these four characteristics.

Non-inflammatory arthritis (osteoarthritis is by far the most common type) may be painful, reflecting joint damage, and swelling is common. However, redness and warmth are absent unless something else, such as infection or bleeding, is also present. And non-inflammatory forms of arthritis are seldom linked to problems elsewhere in the body.

Widespread or Local?

"Widespread" has two meanings. The doctor needs to know not only how many and which joints are affected but also if there is a problem somewhere else in the body that is connected to the joint symptoms.

The greater the number of joints involved, the more likely the problem is to be inflammatory. Symptoms suggesting difficulty in one of the other body systems – the muscles, the skin, the eye, nerves, the lung, heart and kidney – may indicate one of the "systemic rheumatic diseases" – inflammatory conditions such as rheumatoid arthritis and systemic lupus erythematosus.

"Local" means that the problem is confined to joints or nearby tissues. Most non-inflammatory forms of arthritis, and occasionally some inflammatory ones as well, are local, and usually involve only a few joints.

What Is the Pattern of Pain and Stiffness?
How the patient feels at certain times of the day, and for how long, can provide important clues toward a diagnosis. Here are some of the questions doctors ask:

- *How long does it take for you to get loosened up in the morning?*
  "Morning stiffness" refers to the pain and difficulty with movement that patients with inflammation feel upon awakening. It isn't just in the involved joints – it's felt all over. It's in the muscles and in the joints.

  Morning stiffness makes it difficult, even temporarily impossible, to bathe or get dressed. The more activity the person manages, the sooner the problem gets better, but it may take hours to do so. In patients with a major flare-up of arthritis, morning stiffness may continue even all day. Its duration is a pretty good measure of how active the arthritis is.

  Stiffening up – the medical term is "gelling" – after sitting quietly later in the day is a similar symptom. Fortunately, gelling is considerably briefer than morning stiffness.

Non-inflammatory arthritis also has some morning stiffness, but it gets better quickly with activity, usually within
a few minutes.

In contrast to inflammatory stiffness, which improves
with activity, non-inflammatory joint pain gets worse the
more the joint is used. Patients with osteoarthritis of the
hip, for example, are at their worst at the end of the day.

- *How is your energy level?*
Fatigue almost always accompanies inflammatory arthritis. Patients often find it harder to deal with than pain or
stiffness. Among the non-inflammatory forms of arthritis,
only fibromyalgia causes fatigue of similar degree.

- *Do you have pain at night?*
The pain of inflammatory arthritis is often bad at night.
This is particularly true if the spine and the shoulders are
involved. Patients may get to sleep without difficulty, only
to wake in pain in the small hours of the morning. In contrast, patients with non-inflammatory pain generally feel
better with rest.

- *How did it all start, and how has it behaved since then?*
The more sudden the onset of the problem, the more likely
it is to be inflammatory. Gout and polymyalgia rheumatica typically "explode" overnight. Osteoarthritis, however,
may be hardly noticeable at the start. Patients often have
difficulty remembering when it first began.

Non-inflammatory progression tends to be slow and
steady over the years. Symptoms that disappear completely,
only to flare up again later, are indicators of inflammation.

- *Have any joints been warm, red or swollen?*
In clear-cut joint inflammation, there is redness and local
heat in addition to pain and swelling. However, the spectrum ranges from the extreme inflammation of an attack of
gout to, in some cases, a minor puffiness of knuckles in

rheumatoid arthritis. In fact, the entire range of inflammatory signs may be seen at different times in the same patient.

In non-inflammatory arthritis, joint swelling frequently
occurs but clues to inflammation, such as warmth and
redness, are absent. There are exceptions. As already mentioned, infection or bleeding due to injury may mimic
inflammation. In nodal osteoarthritis, a common variant,
warmth and redness may fool the unwary.

- *What's been the response to treatment?*
  As a rule, most of the nonsteroidal anti-inflammatory drugs
  (NSAIDs), such as ibuprofen, naproxen and ASA, are only
  modestly effective in most forms of arthritis. (ASA, or
  acetylsalicylic acid, is also called "aspirin" in the U.S. In
  Canada, "Aspirin" is a brand of ASA.) However, there are
  exceptions, and if a patient describes spectacular improvement in symptoms with treatment, it can help with the diagnosis. For example, patients with inflammatory back pain
  due to ankylosing spondylitis, when started on a regular
  and adequate dose of an NSAID, will suddenly be able to
  sleep through the night. Similarly, the spectacular inflammation of a gouty toe can be wiped out if the right NSAID
  is started at the right time.

Once it is known whether the problem is inflammatory or not,
the next task is to see if the history will lead to a more specific diagnosis. Doctors rely a great deal on what the patient
can tell them about the pattern of the arthritis, any symptoms
in addition to joint pain, the family history and the medication history.

The Pattern of the Arthritis
"Pattern" refers not only to the location in the body, but also
to the behavior of the arthritis. Is just one joint – or are only

a few – the problem? Is the problem mostly in large joints? Is the problem symmetrical, that is, does it involve similar joints on both right and left sides? Are the hand joints involved, and if so, which ones? Does the arthritis come and go, or is it gradually getting worse? Most patterns are not unique to a specific disease, but recognizing a pattern helps to narrow down the possibilities. A few, in fact, are unique, making the diagnosis easy.

Common patterns include:

- Acute monoarthritis – a single joint is suddenly very painful. If this has happened before and the patient is an adult man, chances are this is due to gout or chondrocalcinosis. If this is a first attack, however, infection or bleeding into the joint have to be considered.
- Chronic polyarthritis – persistent involvement of many joints. If just one or two joints are involved, and they are large ones like the knee and the hip, osteoarthritis is a strong bet. If many joints are involved (especially small ones) and both hands are affected, rheumatoid arthritis and nodal osteoarthritis are the most likely diagnoses.
- Spinal pain – both inflammatory (spondylitis) and non-inflammatory (osteoarthritis) problems may cause low back pain, but night pain helps distinguish one from the other.
- Pain felt in muscles – particularly the muscles of the upper arms and the thighs and buttocks – isn't usually caused by muscle inflammation. The problem is more likely to be nearby arthritis, bursitis or tendinitis.

Symptoms in Addition to Joint Pain
In many types of arthritis, inflammation is not confined to joints. As mentioned earlier, other parts of the body may be affected. The rheumatologist then looks for evidence of "systemic disease" – inflammation of other body systems.

Clues to this may be non-specific. Profound fatigue, appetite and weight loss, fever or night sweats are very important symptoms. Or clues may be very specific, and quite helpful in pinpointing the rheumatic syndrome. For example, pleurisy (knife-like chest pain on breathing deeply) may be part of systemic lupus erythematosus, while a man with Reiter's syndrome may report pain on urination and a discharge from his penis.

There isn't an organ system that isn't involved in at least one kind of arthritis – the skin (and hair and nails), the eyes, nose and mouth, the lungs, the heart, the gut, the kidneys and the nervous system. Organ system involvement is not only important for making a diagnosis. It also has important implications for treatment and for the long-term outlook.

Family History of Arthritis
Knowledge that other family members have had arthritis is usually not terribly helpful. Joint problems are very common, and patients seldom know the exact diagnosis of a parent or a cousin. However, some types of arthritis do have a definite tendency to occur in families, and this information can be useful. The best-known example is ankylosing spondylitis. Gout and rheumatoid arthritis also tend to run in families.

Other Drugs Taken
A list of all medications taken, including over-the-counter products, is important. Occasionally, drugs as different as procainamide (for heart irregularities), minocycline (for acne) or diuretics (for blood pressure) will cause serious arthritis problems.

Examining for Arthritis
Many patients are surprised when I ask them to put on a hos-

pital gown. They obviously expect a quick look at the painful area and a diagnosis. I do make "snap" diagnoses, but there is always a risk: arthritis may be the tip of the iceberg, a sign of a condition that affects other parts of the body. If it is, the organ systems involved may provide the clue to the correct diagnosis. A complete physical examination should be the rule.

The General Examination

This examination is particularly important in determining or confirming if there are systemic aspects to the problem.

I ask the patient to strip down to underclothes and slip on a gown. Undressing is important because, in addition to checking blood pressure and testing reflexes, I'm going to be examining the chest, heart and abdomen. In a woman, a breast examination may be necessary. When I do this I try to explain why it's necessary, but sometimes I forget. Here, or in any other part of the examination, the patient should feel free to ask the reasons for the procedure and to request that a friend or partner be present.

The Musculoskeletal Examination

Like the general physical examination, this is tailored to the problem being considered. Someone who has severe low back pain will be examined differently than someone with a painful knee. Nevertheless, a quick survey of the skeleton, taking less than two or three minutes, can give a good idea of what's normal and what's not.

If this quick "screening" picks up a problem, the suspicious area can be more thoroughly assessed.

The physician's sense of feel is important. Touch can detect problems of joint warmth, swelling, crepitus or resistance.

Joint warmth points to inflammation. Usually it refers to a joint being warmer than the area around it, but some joints, the knee especially, are normally cooler than the surrounding tissues. Use the back of your hand to feel the temperature of your kneecap and compare that with your thigh and shin. If the three areas are equally warm, you've got an inflammatory problem with your knee.

Joint swelling may or may not be caused by inflammation. Swelling may reflect fluid within the joint, thickened tissues around the joint, or bony overgrowth around the edges of the joint. If fluid is discovered in the joint, it can be extracted and tested (see Laboratory Tests, below).

Joint crepitus is the term for the grinding sensation that is felt, and sometimes heard, when the joint is being moved. It always means that there's a problem with the tissues of the joint. A good examiner can tell the difference between the crepitus caused by roughened cartilage (the "gristle" at the bone ends), by inflamed synovial tissue (the membrane that lines the joint), or by bone rubbing on bone when the overlying cartilage has been worn away.

Joint resistance, when the physician attempts to move the joint through a full range of movement, may be the first clue to a problem in that joint. This is particularly true in the case of the shoulder, the hip and the back, where pain may be felt some distance from its true source. A good example is hip pain: it's supposed to be felt in the groin, but some patients deny pain there and complain bitterly of pain in the front of

Hand Patterns

The end knuckle of a finger is called the DIP (distal interphalangeal) joint.

The middle knuckle is the PIP (proximal interphalangeal) joint.

The knuckle at the base of the finger is the MCP (metacarpophalangeal) joint.

the thigh, or even in the knee. The knee looks normal, but when the doctor tries to bring the hip up to a right angle and rotate it inward, it just won't go – and the patient repeats that the knee is hurting.

The joints that are involved (as determined by examination) may fit a pattern. This is particularly so in the hands.

- Pattern #1 – a number of DIP joints alone, or in combination with PIP joints, almost always point to nodal osteoarthritis.
- Pattern #2 – a number of MCP joints alone, or more commonly combined with PIP joints, almost always point to rheumatoid arthritis.

Laboratory Tests

The list of tests used in the initial evaluation of the problem is surprisingly short. The lab is being used to address the basic questions: "inflammatory or not?," "systemic or not?"

Later, particularly if a systemic form of arthritis has been diagnosed on the "first pass," more tests may be needed. But if the history and physical examination suggest neither an inflammatory nor a systemic problem, the only reason for further testing is to help to guide treatment.

The following tests are commonly done. The complete blood count (CBC), elevated sedimentation rate (ESR) or C-reactive protein (CRP) and kidney tests are performed most often, to help with diagnosis or to guide treatment. Rheumatoid factor (RF), antinuclear antibody (ANA), joint aspiration and X-rays are done to answer specific questions about diagnosis.

It is important to know that tests can mislead. It's common for a blood test to give a "positive" result for gout, lupus or even rheumatoid arthritis in someone who doesn't have any of these diseases.

Complete Blood Count (CBC)

The complete blood count involves counting the number of red blood cells, white blood cells and platelets – the formed elements of the blood. Some kinds of arthritis, and some kinds of treatment, can affect any or all of the three types.

Since red blood cells carry oxygen from the lungs to the body, white blood cells are one of the body's main means of dealing with infection, and platelets are very important in blood clotting, problems with any one of them may cause real trouble.

- Anemia (a low red blood cell count) is common in inflammatory arthritis. Usually this reflects the fact that the bone marrow, which is where blood cells are made, just isn't able to keep up production when inflammation is present, even if it has all the ingredients, including enough iron. But anemia can also be due to arthritis medicine, particularly NSAIDs such as ASA, which may cause bleeding from a stomach or duodenal ulcer, and a resulting low red blood cell count.

- Low white blood cell counts and low numbers of platelets may occur, separately or together, in some kinds of arthritis. Unfortunately, similar problems may be caused by some of the drugs used to treat arthritis, so the situation can be confusing.

Sedimentation Rate and CRP

The "sed rate" is an old test, but it still has a useful place in medicine. Blood is normally a suspension of cells – red blood cells, mostly. If blood is left to stand in a test-tube, it will separate out – the red blood cells at the bottom, the clear yellow plasma at the top. The speed at which red blood cells settle out (sediment) varies depending on a number of circumstances. Inflammation is one of them. A normal "sed rate" is

20 millimeters per hour or less; in some forms of arthritis it may be as high as 80 millimeters per hour.

A high sedimentation rate can confirm suspicions of inflammation – but, like many other tests, the results may be elevated in conditions other than arthritis, and even in normal people. Nor is the test a good way to follow the course of the disease. To answer the question "Is the patient getting better or worse?" a few questions and a quick exam are far better.

The CRP (C-reactive protein) is a blood test that is starting to be used to replace the "sed rate." It can be automated, so it's cheaper to perform, and it's less likely to be fooled by non-inflammatory conditions than the "sed rate."

Kidney Tests – Blood Creatinine and BUN, and Urinalysis
Kidney problems are usually not evident from the patient's history and physical examination, but are important, because they may be a major complication of some kinds of arthritis. In systemic lupus erythematosus, kidney inflammation may lead to kidney failure. An abnormal urinalysis may point the way not only to the correct diagnosis but also to the correct treatment.

Creatinine and blood urea nitrogen (BUN) are chemical substances excreted by the kidney. In the presence of reduced kidney function, which usually happens without the patient being aware of it, the levels of these chemicals in the blood rise.

Impaired kidney function, not necessarily due to arthritis, is common in older people and in those taking certain medications. Many of the drugs used for arthritis affect the kidneys and, although this isn't usually important, in someone who already has a problem it could be critical. It's vital that treatment not cause already badly functioning kidneys to become worse. To detect patients at risk, these tests are valuable.

Rheumatoid Factor (RF)
This blood test, which detects a protein present in many people with rheumatoid arthritis (RA), is unfortunately neither 100 percent sensitive for everyone with RA, nor specific for it.

In early rheumatoid arthritis, RF will not be detected in at least a third (some think the figure is closer to half) of patients. It is also occasionally found in other forms of arthritis and in some other chronic diseases. Nevertheless, if RF is found in someone whose story and examination are consistent with RA, the diagnosis is basically confirmed.

This test should not be done on anyone with general aches and pains. It should be limited to those who have physical findings consistent with rheumatoid arthritis. This way, the test is not only diagnostic but also tells the doctor something about that person's future (see the chapter on rheumatoid arthritis).

Antinuclear Antibody (ANA)
The ANA is a blood test used in the diagnosis of systemic lupus erythematosus (SLE). As mentioned above, in RA the RF test is negative in a large number of patients in the early stages. But in patients with lupus a negative ANA test is very rare, occurring in 5 percent or less. So a negative ANA reassures the doctor (with about 95 percent certainty) that his or her patient doesn't have that disease. A positive test is not as helpful since it turns up in many normal people, and can be found in quite a number of other diseases as well. In fact, because lupus is relatively rare, it is far more likely that a positive ANA will be a "false" positive rather than a "true" positive.

A positive ANA is just the first step. There must be other proof, from the patient's history, or examination, or from the lab, before SLE can be diagnosed.

Joint Aspiration
This is one test that often turns up the "crucial piece" in the puzzle.

Drawing a specimen of fluid from a swollen joint, using a needle and syringe, and sending it to the lab can supply a great deal of information. Analysis of the white blood cell count helps make the distinction between inflammatory and non-inflammatory arthritis. The fluid can also be tested for infection, and examination using a microscope will show the crystals of gout and chondrocalcinosis if they are present.

Unless the doctor is absolutely certain of the cause, fluid from a swollen joint should always be obtained and examined. This is not as horrible as it sounds since only a small amount of fluid is needed, and this can usually be obtained using a very fine needle. When this is done by an experienced doctor, the discomfort is no more than is felt when a blood sample is taken from the arm.

X-rays and Other Images
In the routine assessment of arthritis, X-rays should be used even less than laboratory tests. They hardly ever help make the diagnosis in patients with recent-onset arthritis. Still, they may confirm suspicions of certain specific problems, such as:

- fractures
- infections involving bone
- cancer involving bone
- chondrocalcinosis, a form of arthritis that involves calcium deposits

They are also used to determine the extent of joint damage, particularly if joint surgery is being considered.

Other ways to look at bone, joints and soft tissues include:

- ultrasound
- bone scans (nuclear isotope scanning)
- magnetic resonance imaging (MRI)
- computerized tomography (CT or CAT scans)

These forms of imaging should be even less frequently used than X-rays. However, they can sometimes provide the critical piece in the puzzle, if done with specific questions in mind.

T W O

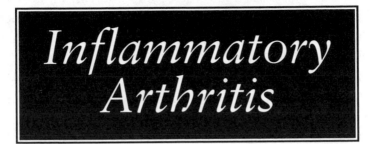

"No-Name" Inflammatory Arthritis

Arthritis is a problem for Kevin, and Kevin is a problem for me. Kevin is a 28-year-old cook. It's clear his problem is inflammatory. For three months now he has had joint pain with typical inflammatory features: swelling, slight warmth, significant and prolonged stiffness first thing in the morning. He has responded fairly well to an NSAID. So far the problem is most obviously in his right knee and both wrists. His fingers are stiff too, but there is no obvious swelling or restricted movement in them.

He has absolutely no other symptoms or physical findings that might help me "pigeon-hole" him. His blood tests have shown a slight anemia, a "sed rate" test result that is mildly elevated and a negative rheumatoid factor. I know that if I X-ray his painful joints I'll simply be wasting money.

I've recommended a trial of hydroxychloroquine, a second-line drug that often helps in a broad range of inflammatory arthritides (that's the plural for arthritis). Kevin is willing to try it, but first he'd like me to answer two simple questions – "What have I got?," and "What's going to happen to me?"

Rheumatologists see a lot of people like Kevin. In fact, just about half of all patients with an inflammatory problem involving multiple joints are initially undiagnosable, despite the doctors' best efforts.

Recent studies have attempted to look at this issue in more detail. Their conclusions are going to help me give Kevin some sort of answer.

First, Kevin is unlikely to have rheumatoid arthritis (RA). We knew that women are roughly three times more likely to get RA, but we now know that for the under-45s the ratio is 6 to 1. Overall, a man's risk of developing RA is estimated at 14 in 100,000 each year, but under 45 the risk is only 2 in 100,000. So, with a negative RF test, RA is very unlikely for Kevin.

In a large American study, patients who, like Kevin, couldn't be given a definite diagnosis at their first visit were followed for several years. In just over half, the problem cleared up completely without a diagnosis ever being made. This is in sharp contrast to those who had clear-cut RA on their first visit. Of those, barely 7 percent were in remission after three years.

Those who didn't clear up were about equally divided into three groups: some developed clear-cut RA, some continued to mystify, and some either went on to more uncommon forms of arthritis (such as lupus) or were felt, in retrospect, never to have had inflammatory arthritis.

The chance of the problem clearing up and going away lessens as time goes by. Kevin has had symptoms for only three months, so he has an almost 60 percent chance of remission. If he had been in trouble for over 18 months, that chance would be only 15 percent.

So Kevin has a lot going for him. He's under 45, his symptoms are recent, his RF test is negative and his rheumatologist can't pin a label on him. This is one time when no diagnosis is a good diagnosis.

Rheumatoid Arthritis (RA)

Sandra is a slender 35-year-old woman who walks with the grace of a professional dancer, which she is. She is also a delight. Her bubbling optimism is infectious and I look forward to her visits.

She first came to me a year ago, when her family physician asked me to see her as soon as possible. She'd been unwell for three months. The slightest effort exhausted her. A month earlier, her knees had become painful and swollen. The PIP and MCP joints of her hands had followed, then her elbows and ankles. To get out of bed and into the shower each morning was extremely difficult. Her whole body was sore and stiff, and only started to improve at mid-morning. Movement and a hot shower seemed to speed the loosening-up process, but later in the day, when she rested and then resumed movement, she re-experienced this stiffness, if only for a few minutes.

Her family doctor had asked her to take eight to twelve ASA a day. He had prescribed the enteric-coated variety, which are coated to protect the stomach. These had helped take the edge off her pain, but had not really affected the swelling.

The lab test results her doctor sent along included:
- a red blood cell count showing mild anemia
- a normal sedimentation rate
- a negative antinuclear antibody test (ANA)
- a negative rheumatoid factor test
- a normal urinalysis
- normal X-rays of hands and feet

Sandra's general physical examination was normal as well. I paid particular attention to her heart and lungs and heard nothing suspicious. I felt for rheumatoid nodules just below the elbow, but found none.

However, the second and third MCP joints of both hands were swollen, as were several PIP joints. I could feel the tension behind the swelling as I pressed firmly with my fingertips; it hurt her, and she told me so. Her wrists and elbows also hurt when I tried to make them bend and extend fully. She hadn't mentioned her feet, but I wasn't surprised when she pulled away as I squeezed the width of her foot at the MTP joints.

At this point, I was reasonably certain that the diagnosis was rheumatoid arthritis (RA). But polyarthritis – that is, arthritis involving many joints – that is symmetrical, particularly in a young woman, can result from other causes such as:

* *systemic lupus erythematosus*

This is the possibility that seems to worry most patients. Young women are commonly the target, and the arthritis in the early stages of SLE may be identical. The fact that Sandra had no symptoms except joint pain and fatigue and had a normal urinalysis was encouraging. The negative ANA test was even more helpful; a negative result is rare in a patient with lupus.

* *psoriasis*

There was no evidence of psoriasis in the usual places – behind Sandra's ears, at the back of her scalp, over her elbows.

* *inflammatory bowel disease*

Similarly, there was no hint of bowel symptoms that might suggest Crohn's disease or ulcerative colitis.

The only thing that made me hesitate to diagnose rheumatoid arthritis was the fact that Sandra's joint symptoms had been present for only a month. Other kinds of joint inflammation can be mistaken for RA – such as the arthritis sometimes seen in measles, hepatitis or parvovirus B19 infection. (Parvovirus is a very common childhood infection. Sometimes an adult who wasn't infected as a child catches it and develops an arthritis that looks a lot like RA but usually clears up in weeks.) We really needed to wait a few weeks to see if things would improve.

I gave Sandra a prescription for naproxen, an alternative to ASA (aspirin), and gave her a follow-up appointment in two weeks. On her return, she felt considerably better. The pain had improved, she was sleeping better and her fatigue was somewhat less. But her swollen joints remained. I arranged for a physiotherapist from the Arthritis Society to see her. I also suggested adding a "second-line" drug to the naproxen, but Sandra wasn't keen on the idea so I didn't press the point.

Two months later, Sandra reported a three-week period when she had no symptoms. Unfortunately, this was followed by a return of all the symptoms, now worse than ever. She was stiff almost until noon each day, and by mid-afternoon she had to lie down and rest because of fatigue. Her joints remained swollen.

At this point, it was clear that more than naproxen was needed, so I added hydroxychloroquine. That was nine months ago. At present, Sandra is experiencing only a few minutes of morning stiffness, but still tires easily. She has a few tender knuckles, but the swelling is gone.

True to her basically optimistic self, Sandra is delighted with her present condition, and has started to press me about when she can stop the medication. I'm a bit more pessimistic. Although her RA is no threat to her as long as it stays at this level, I know from past experience that this may not last.

Rheumatoid arthritis is the most common type of chronic inflammatory arthritis. It can affect any joint, large or small. A dozen or more joints may be affected at any one time. Other parts of the body may be involved in the inflammatory process. Its cause is not known but it is considered to be an autoimmune disease. The immune system, designed to help the body fight off infection, is somehow triggered to react against a patient's own tissues. White blood cells – in particular T lymphocytes – are right in the center of this immune attack. (Doctors have noted that if patients with rheumatoid arthritis are infected with HIV, a retrovirus that causes the T-cell count to drop, their arthritis improves.)

Who Gets Rheumatoid Arthritis?

Rheumatoid arthritis affects at least one out of every 100 North American and European whites. The figure is much lower for Japanese and Chinese and for African blacks, but is the same for North American blacks. In some North American native populations, such as the Chippewa of Minnesota and the Pima of Arizona, it is even higher – about one in 20.

Most women develop RA in their 30s and 40s, most men a few decades later, but in both it can also develop in old age. By age 65 almost 5 percent of women and 2 percent of men will have RA. Roughly three women have RA for every man, but the sex difference tends to narrow with increasing age. For some reason, the prevalence of RA in women (but not in men) has actually gone down over the last 20 years.

RA has a slight tendency to run in families – blood relatives of a rheumatoid arthritic have a risk of about 3 percent instead of the general risk of 1 percent. If one twin has RA, the risk to the other twin is from around 5 to 7 percent (for non-identical twins) to 30 percent (for identical twins).

Although studies of race and family point to the influence of genetic factors, environmental factors must also play a part. In South Africa, for example, one black group has RA much less often than the white population, but only in a rural setting. When these people move to the city, they acquire RA at the same rate as whites.

American College of Rheumatology Criteria for RA

1. morning stiffness of at least one hour
2. arthritis (with swelling) in at least three joint areas (right or left PIPs, MCPs, wrist, elbow, knee, ankle, MTP joint areas)
3. hand-joint arthritis (in at least one of the following: MCP, PIP, wrist)
4. symmetric joint swelling

(Criteria 1 to 4 must be present for at least six weeks)

5. subcutaneous nodules
6. positive rheumatoid factor (RF)
7. typical X-ray changes

If a patient has at least four of these features, the likelihood of the disease being rheumatoid arthritis is much greater than 90 percent.

Using these criteria, at least nine out of ten cases of RA will be detected.

How Is Rheumatoid Arthritis Diagnosed?

We don't know the cause of RA, so we can't identify it by testing for the cause. Instead, we rely on a group of features, or criteria, that fit most patients who are considered to have RA and exclude, as far as possible, those with other kinds of arthritis.

These criteria aren't infallible. There is still a chance that someone who meets the criteria will eventually prove to have something else. But that rarely happens, and treatment tends to be similar in such cases anyway.

Morning Stiffness

This isn't unique to RA. It's seen in many kinds of inflammatory arthritis, and in some (such as fibromyalgia) that aren't inflammatory.

This symptom has never been well explained. It has been suggested that the stiffness is due to fluid accumulating in the tissues around joints when the joints are rested, such as they are overnight. The duration of morning stiffness is a rough guide to how active RA is at any given moment. In very active RA, it may take until noon to loosen up, and a few people insist it never does. In patients who have shown major improvement, morning stiffness may be as brief as five or ten minutes.

Joints Affected

What makes RA different from other types of arthritis is that there are so many affected joints, both large and small, both weight-bearing and non-weight-bearing.

The MCP and PIP joints of the hands are almost always affected. The MCP joints of the index and long fingers are particularly vulnerable. Other kinds of arthritis occasionally affect these two joints, but 95 percent of the time the problem is due to RA.

The MTP joints of the feet are just as commonly inflamed.

Any joint can be affected by RA, however, and in very active disease dozens frequently are. The diagram facing gives an idea of how many joints are involved in RA, and how often. The pattern is usually (though not always) similar on both sides of the body. If one elbow, shoulder or wrist is causing grief, the other usually follows.

Rheumatoid Nodules

These are bumps, from the size of a kernel of corn to that of a small cherry, that develop under the skin. The most typical location is on the forearm, just below the elbow. Pressure seems to trigger their development; habitually resting a forearm on the arm of a chair or on a table is thought to be a factor. Less commonly, people develop nodules over the Achilles tendon (where the back of a high shoe or boot presses), or over knuckles of fingers or toes where pressure is applied again and again.

Nodules may be single or in clusters. Some can be moved about under the skin, while others seem stuck to the underlying bone. They aren't painful unless they are injured or infected. They may be mistaken for other kinds of bumps, including "tophi" (deposits of uric acid), seen in some patients with gout. Very uncommonly, rheumatoid nodules are present by themselves, without any other evidence for RA.

Frequency of RA in the various joints

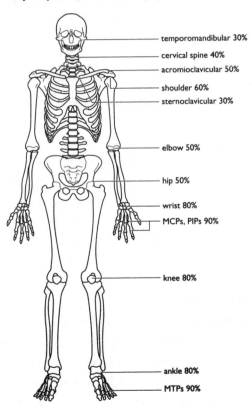

temporomandibular 30%
cervical spine 40%
acromioclavicular 50%
shoulder 60%
sternoclavicular 30%

elbow 50%

hip 50%

wrist 80%
MCPs, PIPs 90%

knee 80%

ankle 80%
MTPs 90%

The exact cause of rheumatoid nodules is not known. There must be some factor beyond local pressure or injury, since nodules appear in less than 20 percent of cases.

In some patients, treatment with methotrexate, even though it helps control joint inflammation, causes the nodule problem to get worse – and we have no idea why.

Nodules that are particularly irritating or unsightly may shrink following corticosteroid injection, and some can only be dealt with surgically. Unfortunately, they often promptly return.

Since almost all patients with nodules have rheumatoid factor (RF) in their blood, RF may be involved in "vasculitis" (inflammation of a small blood vessel) triggered by local injury from pressure. The body may react locally to the vasculitis inflammation, and the attempt at healing may result in a lump of scar tissue below the skin.

Nodules may eventually go away, but they often persist after all other evidence of RA has been suppressed.

Rheumatoid Factor

Rheumatoid factor (RF) is a protein that can be detected in the blood of most patients with RA. It's an antibody – a type of protein that is normally produced to fight off infection. In the case of RF, however, there is no obvious infecting agent, so we don't know what triggers the antibody production. Many different organisms, both bacterial and viral, have been suspected, but convincing evidence for any infectious cause has never been found.

RF is produced by lymphocytes, a type of white blood cell that collects in great numbers in the inflamed joints in rheumatoid arthritics. RF certainly plays a role in the inflammation and the damage in the joint, and elsewhere, that results. Its precise role is under study.

RF is found in the blood of about 60 percent of new cases of rheumatoid arthritis, and these patients are called "seropositives." In general, patients who are "seropositive" right from the beginning are affected much more severely than "seronegatives." As the disease progresses, more and more patients change from "seronegative" to "seropositive." Even then, though, up to 20 percent remain RF negative. It's quite possible that these patients have an entirely different, although very similar, disease.

RF is also found in other diseases, with and without arthritis, and in some normal people. Clearly, rheumatoid factor has a lot to do with RA, but it is not the cause.

X-ray Changes

The most typical change observed using X-rays is an erosion of bone at the margins of a joint. These changes can be seen in any joint that is inflamed long enough. While a few patients are remarkably resistant to this development, 70 percent of those who eventually develop erosions will show the first evidence of this within three years. In fact, one research study showed that this can happen by the end of the first year. This is the main reason why doctors tend to treat RA much more aggressively than they used to. We now realize that it's a lot easier to prevent damage than to reverse it.

How Does Rheumatoid Arthritis First Show Up?

The Sudden, Explosive Onset

Life for Mark, a 56-year-old security guard, was literally transformed over three days. This man who had never taken a sick day was suddenly unable to shampoo his hair, and could barely hold a knife and fork. Almost three dozen joints were swollen and painful – fingers and wrists, shoulders, ankles and toes. Even his left jaw (temporomandibular) joint was affected. He was stiff all day long, fatigued by four p.m., and only managed four hours' sleep at night because of shoulder and wrist pain. His weight had dropped 10 to 15 pounds.

By the time I saw him several months later, two additional pieces of information were available. Testing had revealed a positive rheumatoid factor (RF), and therapy with full doses of naproxen had done absolutely nothing.

Having discussed the issues with Mark, I initiated a program to bring the condition under control as quickly as possible. I substituted prednisone for the naproxen and started him on weekly methotrexate. The prednisone, one of the most powerful anti-inflammatories we have, was for short-term control. The methotrexate would work more slowly, but would eventually allow us to gradually taper off the prednisone entirely.

I saw Mark in follow-up two months later. He told me that after two days of prednisone he had been able to get his dress shoes on for the first time in two months. Except for slight swelling and tenderness in the right ankle, I found nothing on examination. He had no morning stiffness and had gained five pounds. He was back at work. His prednisone had already been lowered to twice daily. I gave him directions for further lowering of the prednisone, and an appointment in eight weeks' time.

RA joint damage: early and late

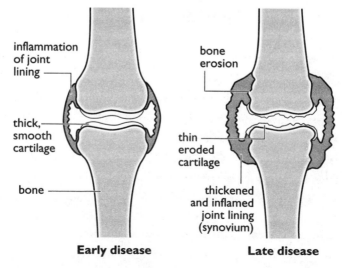

inflammation
of joint
lining

thick,
smooth
cartilage

bone

bone
erosion

thin
eroded
cartilage

thickened
and inflamed
joint lining
(synovium)

Early disease   **Late disease**

Approximately 15 percent of cases will "explode" over a matter of a few days. Although not all the joints that will eventually cause trouble will be involved in this first attack, there will be quite a number – two dozen is typical. They will include both large and small joints, and especially the MCPs and MTPs. Similar joints on both right and left sides will be involved. Morning stiffness and fatigue will be prominent.

The Gradual Onset
But about 75 percent of the time – as with Sandra – the picture is less spectacular. A wrist becomes swollen and for some time it's the only problem. Or a patient develops marked tenderness under the balls of both feet (the MTP joints), particularly when first getting up in the morning. Gradually, over several weeks to several months, more and more joints join the picture. Fatigue and morning stiffness make their appearance. It may take a year or so before the picture is clear enough for a definite diagnosis.

The Gout-like Onset
In 10 percent of cases, RA starts off much like gout. A single joint, such as a knee, wrist or shoulder, suddenly becomes very painful, swollen and warm. Often the pain is so severe that the joint can't be used. Two or three days later, it's back to normal. After a month or so, another attack strikes, usually in another joint. As time goes by, the attacks become more frequent. Gradually they are less and less severe but more and more frequent, and instead of clearing up, the swelling and pain start to persist. One day, perhaps after a year or more, it becomes obvious that we are dealing with RA. This pattern is called palindromic rheumatism, and while it doesn't always turn out to be RA, it most often does.

Julie is a 36-year-old secretary. Nine months before I first saw her, she suddenly developed a very swollen, red and extremely painful left wrist. It felt, she said, as if someone had stuck a knife in it and was twisting the blade. She's right-handed and couldn't think what she had done to provoke this. For three days she had taken acetaminophen with codeine "by the handful" yet had very little sleep, and then, for no apparent reason, the pain and swelling had vanished. Two months later, the same wrist had the same pain and swelling, and the same outcome – gone in three days. One month later it was her right shoulder; for three days she had to use her left hand to brush her teeth. This was followed by three months free of any symptoms, and then her feet began to bother her. Walking, especially first thing in the morning, became very painful. The balls of the feet – the MTP joints – were the problem. Six weeks before I saw her she had developed swelling in several MCP and PIP joints. Pain and stiffness had settled into both hands and wrists. Pain in her shoulders awakened her at night, and her ankles became swollen. She was experiencing severe stiffness until noon, and was profoundly fatigued.

Julie's family doctor had already done blood tests. Rheumatoid factor was present, and there was no question her palindromic rheumatism had evolved into rheumatoid arthritis.

I put her on diclofenac, an NSAID, but knew it wouldn't be enough. She was really hurting, and I wanted to get control as soon as possible. I added methotrexate to the diclofenac, and saw her a month later. She was improved but still had a long way to go. I increased the dose of methotrexate. Today she phoned me. She was apologetic but firm. She had stopped the methotrexate; although I had given her an information sheet on the drug, and discussed it with her, she had read more about it and talked to some friends. She was afraid of what it might do to her in the long run. This fear of medication is common. Lists of side effects, however rare, are frightening. I tried to reassure her, but I didn't push too hard. She has an appointment in two weeks. I expect she will be worse.

Palindromic rheumatism may clear up as mysteriously as it comes on, may continue indefinitely, or, as in this instance, may evolve into very active rheumatoid arthritis, requiring aggressive action.

The Non-joint Onset

Very rarely, RA first appears in an "extra-articular" (non-joint) site, with joint symptoms appearing months later. When it does, it usually takes the form of chest complications, and the patient is usually a man.

A friend and medical colleague asked me to see a patient of his. Oscar was a 45-year-old man who had been admitted to hospital two nights before. Oscar had come in with what we call "pleuritic pain" – a sharp, severe pain in the side of the chest that makes taking a deep breath very difficult. A chest X-ray showed an accumulation of fluid in the space around the lung. The combination of pain and fluid accumulation is usually caused by an infection, but cancer or a blood clot in the lung can do the same thing. A good way of finding the cause is to do a "pleural tap": a syringe is maneuvered between the ribs and into the space around the lungs, and some of the fluid is collected and sent to the lab. In Oscar's case the fluid proved not to be infected, but the sugar content was suspiciously low. This is rare, but my colleague is both well informed and bright. He ordered a rheumatoid factor test and it came out positive. That brought me on the scene.

Oscar by this time was quite comfortable and keen to get on his way. He had absolutely no symptoms of arthritis, so I didn't hold him up. I did, however, book a follow-up appointment. When I saw him two months later he had begun having joint pain, and within another month the diagnosis of RA was clear.

That was fifteen years ago. I treated Oscar with ASA (aspirin) and started him on weekly gold shots, later spaced out to one each month. He's tried to drop the shots entirely on a couple of occasions, but each time his joints flare up. When that happens, I put him back on weekly shots until he settles down and is able to resume the monthly schedule.

I see Oscar about twice a year, to see how he's doing and renew his prescriptions. Visits are in the spring and fall, which fits in with his work. He's a crop-duster, and his work takes him from coast to coast. As far as I know, he hasn't missed a day of work since his hospitalization. If I didn't know he had RA, I certainly couldn't tell by looking at him.

How Is RA Treated?

Rheumatoid arthritis seldom goes away. Eighty percent or more of patients will continue to live with it. When its initial symptoms appear, it's impossible to tell who will do well and who will do badly. **But we do know that joint damage occurs early on, and that we have only a very short period of time – a year or less – to prevent this damage with an effective treatment program.** In practice, this means that treatment is divided into two phases:

- an initial phase (preferably short) where RA is suppressed as completely as possible;
- a long-term surveillance phase where local complications of RA are spotted and dealt with before damage can be caused, and where major flare-ups are anticipated and prevented if possible.

A Long-term Contract

Treatment involves a long-term contract between physician and patient. Each must understand the other as fully as possible. Communications must be open. There will be times when contact is broken off because the disease is stable, but it must be re-established when necessary. And the patient must be able to judge when that time has come.

It's important for the patient to learn as much as possible about the disease, its complications and its treatment. Information can come from many sources – books, others with the disease, other health professionals including pharmacists. The Arthritis Foundation in the U.S. and the Arthritis Society in Canada are valuable sources of information (see Further Resources). Their regional offices contain extensive collections of books, booklets and videotapes, and their websites have a wealth of useful information. They also provide programs for arthritis self-management, and sponsor support groups.

It's also essential to be open and honest with the doctor. If you don't understand something, or you're worrying over something, ask. Doctors often assume that patients know more than they do, while patients are often afraid to appear "stupid." And if you are hesitant to take a medication, or in fact are not taking it – for whatever reason – say so. Your right to refuse treatment is (or should be) recognized by the doctor. The fact that you are refusing shouldn't be taken as a challenge to the doctor's authority, and shouldn't cause him or her to refuse to treat you. There is almost always another way to approach a problem. If the treatment being recommended is truly necessary, more information or changing circumstances will probably enable you to accept it in time.

What Tools Are Available to the Physician?

Treatment can include any or all of the following:

- drugs – NSAIDs, "second-line agents" and corticosteroids
- physiotherapy
- occupational therapy

> ## Five Basic Rules for Treating RA
> * treat as soon as the diagnosis is made
> * treat to suppress all evidence of inflammation
> * fear the disease more than the treatment
> * treat the specific problem in the individual patient
> * use all available resources

* social work
* surgery
* hospitalization
* monitoring the disease

NSAIDs
Nonsteroidal anti-inflammatory drugs are invariably the first class of medication given, and one of the last stopped. They will be described in more detail in the section on drug therapy, but a few generalizations are needed here.

There are a host of drugs in this category, including:

* salicylates (such as enteric-coated ASA)
* ibuprofen
* naproxen
* ketoprofen
* diclofenac
* indomethacin
* tolmetin
* the new COX-2 specific drugs (e.g. celecoxib, rofecoxib)

Whether it's an old-timer like ASA or a relative newcomer like celecoxib, no single drug has ever been shown to be significantly better than another. But different people react differently, with regard to both good and bad effects. This means that a patient may have to try two or three different NSAIDs before deciding which one is best. "Best" may mean "most effective" or "best tolerated." If two drugs are equally good, the choice may boil down to "most convenient" or "cheapest."

No NSAID can completely suppress rheumatoid inflammation. At best, perhaps 25 percent of this problem will be dealt with – just enough to take the edge off. Because NSAIDs have both anti-inflammatory and analgesic (pain-killing) properties, it's sometimes hard to tell which of the two effects is helping the most.

NSAIDs are "base-line" therapy – the first coat of paint. Once it's determined which one seems to be best, which usually takes a few weeks, it's time to add a "second-line" agent, like a second coat of paint over the first. The second-line drug is taken in addition to the NSAID.

Second-line Drugs
These were formerly called "remitting agents," but it's now clear that they don't cause the disease to go away (remit). They can, however, significantly suppress the process. These drugs too are described in more detail in the section on drug therapy.

Older, well-known drugs in this category include:

- hydroxychloroquine
- sulfasalazine
- gold compounds (both intramuscular, given by needle, and oral)
- D-penicillamine
- methotrexate (also known as amethopterin)
- azathioprine

In recent times, a number of others have been added:

- cyclosporin
- minocycline
- leflunomide

- etanercept
- infliximab

All of these drugs help suppress joint inflammation. As with NSAIDs, the discovery of the best one for the individual patient is a trial-and-error process. This doesn't rule out intelligent guesses, because the odds are better for some than for others. At best, a given drug will work well in about two-thirds of all patients, and have no major effect on the other third.

These agents are also called "slow-acting drugs," because it may take up to six months for their full benefit to develop; even the fastest usually takes at least a month. Even if a drug works extremely well initially, as time goes by the benefit may be lost. This happens with all drugs in this class.

For many years, my usual practice was to try one second-line drug after another. If one drug didn't help after several months, or if it initially helped but later lost its effect, I would move on to the next on my list. This was acceptable for many patients, but for others valuable time was wasted; joints were being damaged right under my nose.

There is now proof that combining several second-line drugs (such as hydroxychloroquine, sulfasalazine and methotrexate) results in a better outcome, particularly in patients with very aggressive RA.

Some of the newer agents – such as cyclosporin, leflunomide, etanercept and infliximab – also appear to work extremely well in combination with methotrexate.

In helping a patient choose a second-line drug or drugs, I attempt to calculate how aggressive that person's RA is likely to be, whether the "window" until joint damage begins is fairly wide or just barely open. Relatively mild RA may allow for a leisurely trial of hydroxychloroquine; very painful and extensive RA, particularly in an elderly person with a positive test for rheumatoid factor (RF), calls for one of the stronger agents, alone or in combination.

Finally, for the very severely affected patient, one who has not responded to any of these conventional approaches, research is being done into the effectiveness of bone marrow transplantation. This treatment – which involves destroying the patient's own bone marrow blood cells with drugs, and replacing them with either donated or previously saved bone marrow cells – is essentially the same used in treating some forms of cancer. It is physically very difficult for the patient to undergo, but the hope of a "cure" may make the risk and discomfort worthwhile.

A number of patients with severe autoimmune disease, including rheumatoid arthritis, have been successfully treated, but considerably more remains to be learned. Are there patient characteristics that can predict success or failure? What are the short-term risks of infection and death? What are the long-term risks of the arthritis coming back? Is it possible that the treatment itself may cause cancer?

Corticosteroids

Corticosteroids (also known as glucocorticosteroids or "steroids") are synthetic versions of a hormone that is produced in the adrenal gland. This class of drug has incredibly powerful anti-inflammatory effects, but also has major side effects.

Corticosteroids come in tablets and in injectable forms, which may be given intramuscularly (into muscle), intravenously (into a vein), or intra-articularly (into a joint).

Because of the long-term risks of the oral form, it is wise to avoid it whenever possible. But low doses (5 milligrams or less of prednisone) carry very little risk, and in fact may help protect against joint damage. I use prednisone when the situation calls for it. This is usually when I'm starting a patient on a second-line agent. Steroids can be used as a "bridge" until the second-line agent takes full effect or, later, as a supplement if the effect isn't quite good enough.

High-dose intravenous corticosteroids are sometimes used to provide short-term major suppression of rheumatoid arthritis until long-term treatment (that is, one of the second-line drugs) takes hold.

The risk with intra-articular steroids is very low and the possible benefit very high, particularly if a joint such as a knee is making it impossible for the patient to carry on. Benefits are felt almost overnight and tend to last for a long time.

Physiotherapy, Occupational Therapy and Social Work
A good example of what these professionals have to offer can be found in the chapter on treatment. All are very helpful, particularly:

- to educate the patient about the disease
- to teach the patient how to use joints without causing damage
- to teach the proper role of exercise
- to develop and teach programs to get inflamed joints moving again
- to provide splinting and cushioning to reduce pain and protect joints
- to assess the home and the workplace and recommend changes or tools that will make functioning easier, less painful and safer
- to provide an "early warning" system, particularly if a problem arises that requires a doctor's attention

The goal is to make the patient part of the treatment team. If the general principles of the treatment are incorporated into daily life, the course and the outcome will be much more favorable.

The help of a social worker can be crucial. Once rheumatoid arthritis develops, a number of issues can suddenly become major obstacles to recovery. Problems of short-term and long-term disability, income assistance and job retraining may seem too great to handle. Marriages can buckle under the stress of sudden changes in the patient's occupational, domestic and sexual roles. Depression may make the disease doubly difficult to bear. A social worker can be of great help in discussing these "hidden" issues, and in developing ways to cope.

Surgery
Surgery in RA has come a long way in the last 30 years. There is more extensive comment in the chapter on treatment, but here are some of the procedures used, with greater or lesser success:

- The most common type of surgery in RA is carpal tunnel release. It is generally uncomplicated and very successful.
- Repair of ruptured tendons (almost always the ones that straighten out the fingers) is worthwhile and usually successful. It should be done as soon as possible after the rupture occurs.
- Finger-joint surgery can improve the look of the hand, but usually doesn't improve finger flexibility.
- Surgical replacement of knee and hip joints is usually extremely successful in restoring function and reducing pain.
- Shoulder surgery and foot surgery may help with pain, but are not as successful as knee or hip surgery in getting rid of pain or restoring function.

- Elbow surgery is in a transition phase. A new approach, using a three-part artificial joint instead of the older hinge prosthesis, is very promising for both pain relief and improved function. Whether the new elbow will hold up over time remains to be seen.
- In the past, surgical synovectomy (the cutting out of inflamed joint lining) was often carried out in joints such as the knee. This isn't done much nowadays because (1) the tissue often grows right back, (2) rehabilitation is slow and difficult, (3) infection is a real worry and (4) often the same result can be achieved with the injection of a radioactive form of yttrium, which burns and scars the inflamed lining.

Hospitalization

Admission to hospital, particularly a hospital with a specialized rheumatic disease unit, provides the patient with a number of benefits under one roof at one time:

- respite from the physical demands of the household and workplace
- the opportunity to rest painful inflamed joints
- the skills of a physiotherapist and occupational therapist
- the occasion to learn about the disease
- the opinions of a variety of specialists
- an environment where the effect of treatment can be observed, and treatment adjusted accordingly
- access to a wide variety of diagnostic tests
- assistance in addressing the many social, emotional and occupational challenges posed by RA

Hospital admission is particularly helpful to the patient who has only recently developed the symptoms of RA.

When hospitalization is not a practical option, and often it isn't, therapy and other services may be available on an outpatient basis. Some professionals – in particular physical and occupational therapists, and social workers of the Arthritis Society – assess and treat patients in their homes. Indeed, this is often better than hospital assessment, as specific barriers to restoration of health and function can be identified in the home.

Monitoring the Disease

One of the real problems in treating RA is recognizing when it's time to change the approach. It's too easy to check a patient briefly, mentally compare the status to what it was at the last visit, and continue the same treatment. Instead of words of encouragement and a prescription renewal, the patient often needs a major rethinking. Physicians' memories may be faulty, and patients who are used to feeling bad are often unaware of a slow change for the worse.

It's easy to monitor the progress of some conditions; with hypertension, for example, you simply put on the blood-pressure cuff and take a reading. There have been many attempts to develop a similar "progress test" for RA, but no easy answer has been found.

- X-rays are expensive, expose patients to radiation and record only major damage, after it has occurred.
- The duration of morning stiffness is a crude measurement of how well or poorly the patient is doing, as is the length of time it takes for fatigue to come on each day.
- Blood tests, and especially the sedimentation rate, are too inaccurate to be a basis for treatment decisions. It's true that rheumatoid factor (RF) often becomes negative in remission, but by the time that's detectable even the neighbors know things are better.

- A "joint count" – an inventory of swollen and painful joints – is one way of keeping track over time.
- A number of questionnaires have been developed, and have been shown to reflect very closely the activity of RA. The simplest of these, the HAQ, or Health Assessment Questionnaire, can be completed by the patient in minutes. It can help a great deal in determining whether a treatment is effective, or whether it's time to take a new approach.

What Is the Long-term Outlook?

Ian became my patient 23 years ago. He was a policeman, 29 years old. For a year his sleep had been interrupted by shoulder pain, and he had been limping for the last nine months because of ankle and foot pain. Morning stiffness lasted four hours, but he continued to work. The rheumatoid factor test was strongly positive. I diagnosed RA, even though he hadn't yet had problems with his hands or wrists.

I started Ian on enteric-coated ASA, but he promptly developed a bleeding ulcer. (This can happen with any of the NSAIDs.) Like many people who develop this complication, Ian had no stomach pain to warn him. His stools turned black, standing up made him dizzy and his hemoglobin dropped. I stopped the ASA.

Over the years, Ian has been on many NSAIDs and fortunately has never bled again. He has also been on low-dose prednisone for most of this time. Early on I started him on gold injections and for four years he did very well. Then gold lost its effect on him and I replaced it with D-penicillamine. Once more he did well, with an apparent remission for three years. Over the next seven years his treatment shifted back and forth between D-penicillamine and hydroxychloroquine, and his arthritis came and went. Control was erratic, however, so I switched him to methotrexate. That was seven years ago, and though he still has episodic flares – particularly in his knees, which settle down with cortisone injections – he considers that he is doing pretty well.

But years of rheumatoid inflammation have had an effect. He had to have two tendons in his left hand repaired because long-standing wrist inflammation had caused them to thin and rupture. Both shoulders have had surgery, and the joints have been replaced with metal and plastic. This relieved the severe shoulder pain which was the main reason for the surgery, but the range of movement in his shoulders is still very limited. This type of surgery has a long way to go before it will be as good as knee or hip replacement surgery. Finally, Ian has undergone fusion of two bones in his heel, in a mostly successful attempt to reduce the pain from a very badly damaged joint.

Fortunately, Ian has had a very supportive wife, and very understanding workmates. With modifications, he continued to work in the police department. Within the past year, however, he did retire. He probably could have stayed on, but he was experiencing more and more pain in previously damaged joints. Now that he has stopped work, he has much less pain and fatigue. He has a bit of difficulty carrying out almost all activities of daily living – such as getting out of a bathtub and washing his hair – but there is really nothing he can't do.

The progress of rheumatoid arthritis is unpredictable, but effective treatment does help slow the deterioration. In a minority of cases, there is total remission.

The outcome is likely to be poorer if rheumatoid factor (RF) is present from the beginning; if there are rheumatoid nodules; and/or if the patient is over age 60 when the disease first appears. However, the type of onset (sudden, gradual, gout-like or non-joint) is *not* an indicator of how the disease will progress.

The "worst case" scenario is represented by a study from England. Doctors there looked back at 112 patients who had first been seen between 1964 and 1966. After 20 years:

- a third were dead
- a fifth were severely disabled
- a fifth were leading a normal life
- almost a quarter had had major reconstructive orthopedic surgery

A similar study was done in Canada, in which 681 out of an original group of 1,043 were available for follow-up after an average of 12 years:

- a quarter had died
- at the beginning, half of the patients were leading a normal life
- at the end, 17 percent were leading a normal life
- 16 percent were completely disabled
- 10 percent had no disability

Several important points should be made. First, although most of the deaths were not obviously related to RA or its treatment, there was nevertheless a greater mortality rate than expected. And, second, treatment with second-line drugs had been delayed, on average, over 10 years from the time that RA had been first diagnosed.

Two recent studies point to a more optimistic outlook.

One, from Finland, reported on 103 patients who had had RA for an average of 16 years.

- 23 percent had completely normal function
- only 6 out of 103 could be considered very severely disabled
- 20 percent had total joint replacement of knees or hips

Another Canadian study looked at a group of 128 RA patients over a somewhat shorter time frame – 6.5 years on average:

- 42 percent of patients had experienced RA continuously
- 40 percent had arthritis that came and went
- 18 percent had experienced only one attack

Despite the fact that 80 percent still had some ongoing difficulty, a third had no joint swelling; a quarter had no evidence of damage showing up on X-rays; and almost a third were functioning completely normally.

The major difference between these recent studies and the two earlier ones is that, while the observation periods were admittedly shorter, in the majority of the recent patients, **treatment with second-line drugs was started within three years of their first symptom.**

We have learned how devastating a disease RA can be, and we have learned that its damage frequently occurs early. We have also learned to be comfortable with second-line drugs. Drugs like gold and methotrexate have moved from being "last resort" to being "first resort."

Unfortunately, some patients are still more afraid of the treatment than the disease, and shy away from second-line drugs. If the initial presentation of the disease suggests a milder course, this may not make much difference. But when the markers for more severe RA are present, patients need to understand the damage that may be done if second-line treatment is delayed.

Inflammatory Arthritis of the Spine and Extremities

This is a family of conditions that includes psoriatic arthritis, ankylosing spondylitis, the arthritis of inflammatory bowel disease, and reactive arthritis (Reiter's syndrome).

Rheumatologists refer to this family as "seronegative spondylarthritis." "Seronegative" simply means that the blood test for rheumatoid factor is negative, and "spondylo" is a prefix that means "spine."

Members of this family share a variety of distinguishing characteristics:

- a unique pattern of spinal and extremity arthritis
- inflammation of ligaments and tendons
- occasional inflammation of the eye and heart
- psoriasis in some
- evidence of an inherited predisposition

Compared to rheumatoid arthritis, this pattern of arthritis is likely to involve fewer joints, involve joints asymmetrically, so that the "twin" (such as the opposite knee) of an inflamed joint is not affected, and involve the lower spine, particularly the sacroiliac joints.

Inflammation of ligaments and tendons, particularly where they attach to bone, is common and characteristic. The attachment points, in medical jargon, are "entheses," and common sites of quite painful "enthesitis" include the back of the heel, where the Achilles tendon attaches, and the underside of the heel, where inflammation may produce a "heel spur."

Inflammation of eye and heart tissues may also occur in these forms of arthritis, although this is fortunately infrequent. Eye inflammation is usually obvious, with redness and discomfort, and should be assessed by an eye specialist. Heart-tissue inflammation may result in a leaky aortic valve (so that blood leaks back from the main blood vessel, the aorta, into the heart) or in abnormal conduction of the electrical impulse that stimulates heart muscle contraction.

Psoriasis, a chronic inflammatory disease of the skin, can

accompany at least two members of the family – psoriatic arthritis and Reiter's syndrome.

Psoriatic Arthritis (PsA)

Jim is a 31-year-old chiropractor with psoriatic arthritis. His hands are his livelihood. He has had psoriasis for 10 years. Because the rash is tucked away behind his ears and in the hair at the back of his scalp, not many people are aware of it. A close look at his fingernails, though, shows the telltale indicators. One is an accumulation of thick yellow debris lifting and irregularly separating several nails from their underlying beds. The other is the finely pitted appearance of many of his nails, as if a fine needle had pricked the surface, leaving dozens of tiny little pits in each nail.

Common sites of foot pain

Achilles tendon (tendinitis)

MTP joints (metatarsalgia)

Plantar fascia attachment at heel (plantar fasciitis)

Over the last four years the arthritis, which in his case involves mainly the end joints of his fingers (the DIP joints), has given him more and more concern. First one, then another, and now three of the end knuckles in each hand have become swollen and red. When the first one came on, it looked so inflamed that his family doctor put him on antibiotics, mistaking the arthritis for an infection. These knuckles are sore too, but not as painful as they look.

And it isn't just Jim's fingers. One by one, several of his toes swelled and became tight and shiny – what rheumatologists call "sausage toes." There were two toes affected on one foot, three on the other.

Generally, Jim gets by. He has some difficulty with fine finger movements such as buttoning and tying shoelaces and finds it is difficult to open a milk carton. But before coming to see me, he hadn't bothered taking the NSAIDs his doctor had prescribed. He probably wouldn't have come except for two new developments – a tender right knee and a painful left thumb MCP joint. His arthritis had finally gotten his attention.

My examination confirmed the psoriatic changes in his scalp – fine silvery scales covered reddish irregular patches – and in the nails. The finger and toe redness and swelling were obvious. When I checked the knee, though, it was clear that the joint itself was not inflamed. The problem was with the tendon below the kneecap. It was very tender, particularly where it attached to the bone of his upper shin.

I prescribed an NSAID, in this case naproxen. My plan now is to see how Jim responds. I expect that he'll feel a significant lessening of his symptoms, but that the inflammation will persist. If that is so, and if he agrees, I plan to add a second-line drug, in this case sulfasalazine.

What is Psoriatic Arthritis?

Psoriatic arthritis (PsA) is the arthritis linked to psoriasis. Although it has been around for years, it was only 30 years ago that rheumatologists finally agreed that it wasn't just another type of rheumatoid arthritis (RA), but was unique.

One reason for the confusion is that PsA shows up in a number of different ways, one of which looks very much like rheumatoid arthritis. Another is that it wasn't really until 50 years ago that modern medicine began to look closely at arthritis in general. When that happened, people started to notice the differences in many kinds of arthritis, not just PsA. And this process of "discovering" new kinds of arthritis isn't over yet.

Who Gets It?

You have to have psoriasis to get PsA. Psoriasis is a very common chronic skin condition; it occurs in 1 to 2 percent of Caucasians. We don't know what causes it, but inheritance plays a big role. Children of a parent with psoriasis are three times more likely to have psoriasis; if an identical twin has psoriasis, there is a 75 percent chance the other twin will have it too. Its typical appearance is that of a reddish patch of skin covered with a silvery or yellowish scale. These patches are of all sizes, and irregular in outline. They tend to occur over pressure points such as the knees and elbows. They are equally common in the scalp, behind the ears, or in the navel. In fact, psoriatic plaques can be anywhere. They may be numerous, covering almost all skin surfaces, or found only after a careful search. They may come and go, and when they go the skin may regain its normal appearance.

As in Jim's case, psoriasis may affect the nails. This happens in just under half of all people with psoriasis (although the nails are involved in almost 90 percent of PsA patients).

About 10 percent of people with psoriasis develop PsA. If a careful X-ray search for evidence of arthritis is made (particularly if the sacroiliac joints at the base of the spine are X-rayed), this number can be pushed up to around 40 percent, but most of the extra 30 percent won't have symptoms.

Although psoriasis may start at any age, commonly in the late teens, the arthritis usually makes its appearance later – about equally in the 20s, 30s and 40s. I've said that you have to have psoriasis to get PsA. This isn't absolutely true, because

> ## Signs and Symptoms That Suggest Psoriatic Arthritis
> * psoriasis
> * redness and swelling at end knuckles
> * swollen, inflamed fingers and toes
> * tendinitis and enthesitis
> * back pain

in a small number of people (possibly as much as 15 percent) the arthritis shows up first. The usual story, though, is that the skin rash has been present for a number of years, or (less often) that the rash and the arthritis develop together.

Finally, and this is very different from RA, the numbers of men and women with PsA are about equal.

What Are Its Characteristics?
PsA has a number of distinct features. In some patients one feature may dominate, in others, another. Features may be present in varying combinations, and the pattern may even change with time, so that the emphasis shifts.

Characteristics that suggest PsA include the following:

Redness and Swelling at the Ends of the Fingers
This is due to arthritis of the end knuckles (DIPs), and was the prominent feature of Jim's hand inflammation. Inflammation of DIP joints is uncommon except in three instances – PsA, nodal osteoarthritis and (very rarely) gout. But in PsA the swelling and redness tend to involve the surrounding tissue as well as the joint. Not all DIP joints become inflamed, and those that do often develop the condition in sequence rather than all together.

Swollen, Inflamed Fingers and Toes
This too happened to Jim. Here the inflammation is not confined to the joints – it spills over into the surrounding tissues.

When I see fat, red "sausage" toes, I start to look for evidence of psoriasis. Such inflammatory swelling of an entire finger or toe (called "dactylitis") is almost always due to inflammation of the finger tendon, and in most cases that means psoriatic arthritis.

Tendinitis and Enthesitis
"Entheses" are the points where ligaments and tendons attach to bone. Pain due to inflammation at an enthesis is very common in everyday life; "tennis elbows" and "heel spurs" are two examples. But in PsA, tendinitis and enthesitis are even more common. In Jim's case, the location was a bit unusual – where the tendon from the kneecap attached to the upper shin. Much more commonly, the inflammation involves either the Achilles tendon where it attaches at the back of the heel, or the underside of the heel itself. This last location is where the tough tissue that protects the sole of the foot (the "plantar fascia") attaches to the heel.

Back Pain
Most people with psoriasis don't have back pain, but if they do it's identical to that of ankylosing spondylitis (AS). This type of back pain is characteristically worse at night, often awakening the patient, and first thing in the morning. As the patient becomes more active, the stiffness and soreness gradually lessen. There is another similarity to AS when PsA involves back pain – those affected are more than twice as likely to be male. This is quite unlike the equal sex distribution in other forms of PsA.

How Is It Diagnosed?
Diagnosis is easy if psoriasis co-exists with several red, swollen DIP joints, a swollen pink finger or toe, or a swollen knee, ankle or wrist.

In general, patients with PsA test negatively for rheumatoid factor (RF).

How Is PsA Treated?

Despite the fact that we spend considerable time separating PsA from RA, the treatment of the two is almost identical:

- oral anti-inflammatory drugs (NSAIDs)
- second-line agents (such as sulfasalazine, methotrexate and cyclosporin. Some of the newer drugs – such as etanercept – also look promising)
- corticosteroids by injection into inflamed joints, and occasionally by mouth
- occupational therapy and physiotherapy
- surgery, when indicated

What Is the Long-term Outlook?

Two individuals I have come to know well over the years have had quite different experiences with psoriatic arthritis.

When I first saw Margaret a decade ago she was 46, the mother of two and a physician. She came to me with the following story. Psoriasis, mainly over the elbows and the back of the scalp, had developed when she was 21. At 34 she had a severe bout of neck pain for several months, and two years later an episode of severe right foot pain that also lasted several months. Its location, deep in the pad of tissue under the heel, as well as her recollection that it was very painful first thing in the morning and became bearable only after several hours of limping, convinced me that this was an enthesitis – in this case "plantar fascitis," or inflammation of the plantar fascia.

Six weeks before her first visit to me, the knuckle at the base of Margaret's right index finger (the 2nd MCP) had swollen, turned red and become painful. Aside from scalp psoriasis, and pitting of several nails, my examination turned up nothing of note. She had already started on naproxen and felt somewhat better, and I elected to keep her on it.

Over the next decade, she averaged three or four visits a year. Each visit would be provoked by something new happening – often the swelling up of one or two knuckles, with redness and pain.

In Margaret's case, the DIP joints have only rarely been inflamed – it is usually individual MCPs and PIPs. The swelling and pain tend to gradually cool off after two or three months. In only one case – the right ring finger PIP joint – has the inflammation caused any damage. In that case, the finger became "stuck" in the slightly bent position. An X-ray showed no bone or joint damage; the problem is scarring of the ligaments and tendons around the joint. It is clear that, unlike RA, in PsA these structures are actively involved in the local inflammation. The spread of inflammation outside the joint itself is also probably why psoriatic joints so often look red, quite unlike those in RA.

On a half-dozen occasions, the visit was provoked by inflammation of individual finger tendons. This made bending the fingers to grasp an object, or make a fist, very painful and difficult. Sometimes, in fact, the swelling and pain would be so bad that the finger couldn't be bent at all. This problem usually melted away after I injected the swollen tendon sheath with a corticosteroid.

Once Margaret had a recurrence of her neck pain for several months, and another time she again experienced severe pain under her right heel. Twice her posterior tibial tendons (located on the inside of the ankle, just behind and below the bony "bump") swelled. On several occasions she developed a fat pink toe, a different one each time. Walking was painful, so I had her shoes fitted with molded cushioning insoles until the inflammation went down.

And it did go down each time, usually within two or three months. She has been taking various NSAIDs – indomethacin, piroxicam, naproxen – and they help with each flare-up. Unfortunately, she also gets severe "gut-grief" with them, and has to take misoprostol (a stomach-protector). Eight years ago I started her on hydroxychloroquine and it seemed to reduce the frequency and intensity of her attacks. Three years ago I added yet another second-line drug, sulfasalazine, and I think she has done even better. I last saw her 18 months ago. She had just experienced a flare of inflammation of her right index finger DIP joint, her left index flexor tendon and her left wrist. At my instruction she had taken a brief course of oral prednisone, and had settled down nicely. There was little evidence of inflammation anywhere. I asked her to increase the sulfasalazine dose slightly. It must have worked, or her PsA is taking a holiday, because neither she nor her doctor has asked me to see her again.

Margaret represents one end of the spectrum. Doug represents the other.

Doug was 47 when I first saw him eight years ago. Psoriasis had appeared when he was 37, and arthritis just three months before his visit. Within the span of these three months his right forefoot, at the base of the toes, had swelled and become red and painful. Three toes of his left foot had swelled, and his right knee was twice its normal size and painful. This was followed by pain under his heels that made it even more difficult to walk. He was forced to take sick leave from his foreman's job at GM Diesel.

The intervening years have not been good. Doug hasn't

returned to work. His feet have never resolved completely, and both hands, wrists, elbows and shoulders, as well as his right knee, have become inflamed, gotten better and worse, but never entirely cleared up. X-rays of his hands show erosions in several PIP and DIP joints, as well as the wrists. The toes show similar damage, and there are heel spurs. His grip strength, measured by squeezing a rolled blood-pressure cuff, is 110 with the right hand and 160 with the left (almost anyone without hand arthritis can achieve 300). He can do most things, but with a fair amount of difficulty.

Doug's gradual deterioration isn't for lack of trying. He has been faithful in taking whatever I've prescribed, but unfortunately he has experienced limiting side effects with most drugs. Nausea and vomiting are the most frequent, especially with the two agents I've found to be most effective, methotrexate and azathioprine. Right now he's on intramuscular gold injections. They don't seem to be causing any problems, and he has shown definite slowing of the inflammatory process over the last year.

In general, while PsA causes long-term disability in some, this happens less frequently than in patients with RA of similar duration. Nevertheless, after 10 years of PsA at least 15 percent of all patients are severely disabled. Probably an equal number of patients, if not more, are in remission except for residual damage.

The same sort of treatment philosophy described for RA should hold equally for PsA. Since the outcome in each individual can't be predicted, each person should be treated as aggressively as possible from the very beginning.

Distinguishing PsA from Rheumatoid Arthritis
Psoriatic arthritis may look very much like rheumatoid arthritis. For that matter, some people with psoriasis have RA – after

Rheumatoid Arthritis versus Psoriatic Arthritis

	PsA	RA
involvement of similar joints on opposite sides of the body	uncommon	usual
involvement of DIPs	common	rare
inflammation with joint redness	common	uncommon
number of joints	fewer	more
enthesitis	common	rare
rheumatoid factor	in less than 5 percent	in approximately 80 percent
rheumatoid nodules	absent	present in 20 percent
sex ratio	equally affected	three times more common in females

all, both psoriasis and RA affect at least one percent of the population, so it would be surprising if they didn't occur together. More often, though, one is confused with the other because both may involve the hands, and in particular the MCP and PIP joints. The diagnosis often rests on such features as the presence of rheumatoid factor and the changes seen in X-rays.

I was recently asked to see Anna because of this very problem. Five months before, she had experienced an explosive progression of pain, stiffness and (in the case of her arms and legs) swelling. The inflammation marched from her neck to her shoulders, and from there to her hands, wrists, elbows, knees, ankles and feet. Morning stiffness was prolonged and severe. Anna was 46 and was an executive assistant in a law firm, but had been unable to work since the episode had begun. Not only that, but she had real difficulty with such basic acts as attending to her personal hygiene.

Both wrists, as well as the majority of MCP and PIP joints in both hands and both right and left MTP joints, were swollen and/or painful.

According to criteria set by the American College of Rheumatology (see preceding section on RA), Anna had rheumatoid arthritis – a persisting inflammatory symmetrical arthritis involving hands and wrists as well as at least one other area, linked to morning stiffness.

But there were other features that indicated PsA. These included both right and left "tennis elbows" as well as tenderness at the point on the right heel where the Achilles tendon attaches. In other words, Anna had enthesitis. She was also seronegative; her rheumatoid factor test had been consistently negative.

The most convincing evidence came from the past. She had been troubled with psoriasis as a teenager, although the only evidence for it currently was in her fingernails. In her early 20s,

---

The Frequency of the Various Patterns of PsA:

- 5 percent to 10 percent look like Jim – primarily showing inflammation of the end knuckles of fingers and toes

- 5 percent have low back pain dominating

- 20 percent look like Margaret, with episodes of inflammation in relatively few joints in an asymmetrical pattern

- 70 percent have persisting inflammatory polyarthritis, most like Doug, with characteristics of PsA, or, much less often, like Anna, whose arthritis is very similar to rheumatoid arthritis.

and continuing until the present flare-up, she had experienced
periodic episodes of single joint inflammation that would
persist for several months and then fade away. A number of
DIPs and MCPs, as well as a wrist and a knee, had been the
targets. This, then, was the background for her current flare-up
– most unlike RA, but quite typical of PsA.

Ankylosing Spondylitis (AS)

Mike is 32 years old and works as a warehouse foreman for a
department store. He was somewhat reluctant to come to see
me. He had been living with his problem for so long that he felt
there was probably little that could be done for it.

Mike was in his early 20s when his back pain started. He
had twisted his back doing some heavy lifting and assumed this
was the cause. But when I heard his description of the pain, it
was so typical that I felt it couldn't be anything but inflammatory. As he said, "Nights are the pits." He awakened regularly,
around three a.m. each night, with a deep, aching pain that
went from the small of his back down into his buttocks.
Rolling over caused intense pain, and getting up out of bed
each morning was an ordeal. He had to work himself into a
sitting position, then slowly stand. The stiffness would gradually wear off by noon, and throughout the rest of the day, as
long as he was active, he had no pain. It was only in the
evening, getting up after watching television, that he was
reminded of the misery of the night to come.

Over the years Mike's back pain had come and gone. There
would be months when he wouldn't even think of it. But for
the last two to three years it had been constant, and it was
getting worse.

I asked the usual questions. Mike had never had psoriasis, or
problems with diarrhea or with a discharge from his penis.
However, he did recall seeing an eye specialist five years before,
when one eye became red and painful. That got better with

treatment and had never recurred. The other clue that I thought significant came up when I questioned him on other members of his family. It turned out that I had seen his mother, many years before, for a very swollen and painful ankle. When I later looked at my notes on her, I noticed that the ankle had settled down after several months, and that I hadn't been able to make a diagnosis. Maybe I could now.

When Mike stood, he had a slightly round-shouldered appearance, and the hollow in the small of his back was straight instead of curved. I measured his chest expansion with a tape measure. It was half of what one might expect. There was a similar shortfall when I measured the movement of his lower spine as he bent forward.

Mike's family doctor had made my job easy. He had ordered a sedimentation test, and the rate was markedly elevated at 55 milligrams per hour. X-rays had been taken of Mike's pelvis and lumbar spine; the lower two-thirds of the sacroiliac joints were partially fused, and several vertebrae showed bony spurs that looked as if they were trying to bridge the gap between them. Finally, although I certainly didn't need it to make the diagnosis, the family doctor had ordered a blood test for HLA (Human Leukocyte Antigen)-B27, and it was positive.

I spent quite a bit of time with Mike, explaining the nature of the problem and the role of treatment. I started him on indomethacin, an NSAID, and arranged for a physiotherapist to show him a program of flexibility exercises.

I've seen Mike once since. The indomethacin hadn't given him heartburn, a possible side effect, and had given him a full night's sleep for the first time in years. He still had morning stiffness, but it was much more tolerable. His main problem was fatigue. My measurements of his chest and back movements indicated approximately 30 percent improvement. He was faithfully doing his exercises and had joined the Spondylitis Association.

AS is the most common type of inflammatory spinal arthritis ("spondylitis" means inflammation of the spine). In extreme cases AS goes on to become "ankylosis" – that is, the normally flexible spine is transformed, because of persisting inflammation, into a rigid calcified column.

This member of the seronegative arthritis family is characterized mainly by inflammation of the spine, and only occasionally exhibits arthritis of the extremities. Psoriasis is absent, but some of the uncommon seronegative features – such as eye and heart inflammation – are occasionally seen.

Who Gets AS?

AS occurs in 0.1 to 0.2 percent of whites (about one-tenth to one-fifth as often as rheumatoid arthritis). It's rare in blacks, but much higher in some native North American groups. Men are three times as susceptible as women. It can occur at any age, but the peak onset is in the late teens and twenties.

The 0.1 to 0.2 percent figure is probably a minimum, because it's based on examination of patients who were admitted to hospital. It's likely that there are many more cases, milder and undiagnosed, outside of hospital. In fact, one Norwegian study turned up a frequency of just over one percent, and only about one-fifth of these had ever been diagnosed! This may mean that AS is as common as RA.

What Are the Characteristics of AS?

Back Pain with Inflammatory Features
This story is so typical that, assuming the doctor has time to listen to the patient, it should never be missed. Pain develops slowly, over months. The pain is so slow and insidious, in fact, that commonly several years go by before the diagnosis is even thought of.

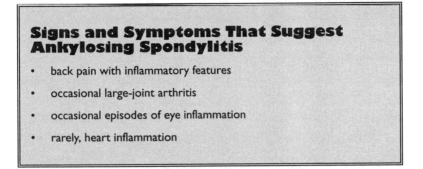

Signs and Symptoms That Suggest Ankylosing Spondylitis

- back pain with inflammatory features
- occasional large-joint arthritis
- occasional episodes of eye inflammation
- rarely, heart inflammation

The pain is "rest pain" and comes on when the patient is sleeping. It is at its worst when the patient tries to move after being still for a while. It's made better by activity, often to the point where it's forgotten. It's often helped a great deal by NSAIDs.

All of this is in contrast to mechanical back pain, which is what common, garden-variety low back pain is called. The pain there comes on suddenly and is made much better by rest; NSAIDs do very little, and activity is associated with increased awareness of pain.

Inflammatory low back pain can be "referred" to (i.e., experienced in) the buttocks or even the upper backs of the thighs. Sometimes pain can be felt elsewhere in the spine – in the neck, or between the shoulder blades. Chest pain, occasionally in the front in the area of the breastbone (the sternum), or coming around the sides of the chest from the back, is frequent, and can be quite severe. All these types of pain, like the low back pain, can be linked to enthesitis (inflammation at the site where ligaments and tendons attach to bone).

In AS, the inflammation is targeted on the spine and sacroiliac region of the pelvis, where the spinal ligaments and muscles are attached. This inflammation causes the pain, and also results in a very unusual form of reaction to inflammation. Unlike rheumatoid arthritis, where inflammation leads to erosion of bone, here new bone growth is stimulated by the inflammation.

Bony spurs grow out from the vertebrae of the spine at the sites of inflammation, tracing the course of the ligaments as they pass up and down to adjacent vertebral bones. In extreme cases, these bony spurs completely bridge the gap between vertebrae, making movement impossible. If this happens throughout the spine, the individual stands and moves rigidly, unable to stand completely erect and unable to turn the head from side to side.

We rarely see AS sufferers end up as "poker spines" nowadays. Some experts believe that this is because NSAIDs help suppress the actual damage as well as "cool off" the inflammation. It's certainly true that before the 1950s – when phenylbutazone, the first truly effective drug for AS, became available – a bent, inflexible spine was accepted as an inescapable result of the disease.

Occasional Large-Joint Arthritis
This may happen in up to 20 percent of people with AS. Hips and shoulders are the most common targets, usually in pairs. Single-joint inflammation tends to be in a knee or an ankle, and tends to be transient. Sometimes a jaw joint is affected, but usually the joint is in the hip or leg. Interestingly, hip-joint inflammation seems to occur only in those who develop AS as teenagers, and then within the first 10 years of the disease. It's very unusual to have someone in his or her 30s or older get hip involvement.

Differences Between Men and Women
In addition to the disease being less frequent in women (especially in the teen years), there are other differences. Women tend to have even more insidious back symptoms, and rest

pain is less severe. On the other hand, it's much more common for women to develop arthritis in arm and leg joints, both at the beginning and later. Looking back, I think this was true in the case of Mike's mother. When I first saw her, ankylosing spondylitis was the furthest thing from my mind. In this I was undoubtedly blinded by the fact that she was a woman; at that time we thought AS was almost always a male disease. But it's also probable that her back symptoms were minimal and she didn't think twice about accepting them as "normal."

Eye Inflammation

Attacks of iritis (inflammation of the iris) occur at some time in up to 25 percent of individuals with AS. One eye becomes red and sore. Vision is blurred and bright lights are painful. The attack subsides over weeks to months, but because the inflammation may leave scars in the area of the pupil, it's wise to see an eye specialist. Local treatment, and often long-term follow-up, may be important to avoid serious trouble later on.

Heart Inflammation

Inflammation of the aortic ring – the tissue where the aortic valve attaches to the heart – may cause scarring and a consequent leaky valve. Because the electrical "cable" that conducts the heartbeat is nearby, scarring can also cause a block in this impulse. It sounds terrible, and I spent a lot of time listening to hearts of people with AS before I realized that this is a very rare event; I've seen it maybe twice in 30 years. The statistics say that it happens in about 5 percent of people with AS.

How Is AS diagnosed?

The most important clue to the diagnosis is the story of night pain and severe morning stiffness that improves significantly as the day goes on. Except in very early cases,

What Is HLA-B27, and What Does It Tell Us?

HLA stands for Human Leukocyte Antigen, meaning an antigen (protein) carried on the outside of white blood cells. The specific antigens we carry are inherited. These complex molecules are important in defending the body against infectious bacteria and viruses and other "intruders."

In the early 1970s it was found that although one particular HLA, called B27, was found in only a small proportion of the population (about 10 percent among Western Caucasians), it was present in most people with ankylosing spondylitis (AS).

B27 isn't the only risk factor for AS, and most people with B27 don't develop the disease. But if one member of a family has AS, the risk for other family members who carry B27 increases to 20 percent. And people who develop AS without carrying B27 usually have milder cases starting at an older age.

The importance of the discovery of the HLA-B27 linkage to ankylosing spondylitis lies in the questions it has raised about the ultimate causes of arthritis. Here is an inherited factor, a marker for arthritis, that is intimately involved in the body's defense against infection. Armed with the knowledge that another B27-linked form of arthritis – reactive arthritis – can be triggered by a number of different infections, researchers are attempting to determine how this comes about. And because both systemic lupus and rheumatoid arthritis also have inherited, and HLA, associations, the answer to that question may be the key to understanding many different kinds of arthritis.

physical examination may show that the spine and chest don't move normally, as in Mike's case. But this lack of movement doesn't necessarily mean that bony bridges have already formed; inflammation itself will interfere with movement. A good or excellent response to NSAIDs completes the picture.

The problem arises when the patient doesn't quite fit this pattern – usually because the response to treatment isn't as dramatic as expected.

Unfortunately, plain X-rays may not show any abnormality for up to 10 years after the symptoms start, and nuclear isotope bone scans are often untrustworthy in AS. If a patient believed to have AS is not responding to the usual treatment, then a CT scan is the best way of determining if there is sacroiliac damage. If positive, treatment should be pursued more aggressively; if negative, the patient's problem should be re-evaluated to see if there is an alternative explanation for the symptoms.

Blood tests, and in particular the test for HLA-B27, are no help. A positive test for HLA-B27 is at least 10 times more likely to be a false positive than a true positive.

Fortunately, most cases do fit the pattern, so there is usually no problem with diagnosis.

How Is AS Treated?

Non-steroidal Anti-inflammatory Drugs
NSAIDs usually make a big difference in AS. Unlike rheumatoid arthritis, where NSAIDs only "take the edge off," in AS relief can be virtually total.

Phenylbutazone was the first of the NSAIDs available. It's still one of the most effective, but because it can cause aplastic anemia (an often fatal condition where the body stops making blood cells) it is usually used only in those rare instances where all the other NSAIDs have failed.

Indomethacin was the next NSAID available. It's quite effective, but because it can cause severe headaches when first taken the patient is usually started on a fairly low dose and gradually worked up to a dose that controls AS symptoms. There is a slight risk of aplastic anemia with indomethacin, but it is rare.

Almost any of the NSAIDs on the market today is effective, but adequate doses must be used. The inflammation of AS tends to "cycle"; that is, at times it will be relatively little and cause problems only at night and briefly in the morning.

Patients should adjust the schedule of their pills to the disease; if symptoms are at a very low level, a single bedtime dose of medication may do the trick. Indomethacin is available in a sustained-release form that gives 12-hour coverage, so it's particularly useful in this situation. Sometimes symptoms improve so much that regular NSAIDs are not needed.

After a period of time, many patients find that their NSAID seems to lose its effectiveness. If they give that NSAID a rest and switch to another for a month or two, they usually find that the original medication, when begun again, is just as effective as it was initially.

Second-line drugs
These have not proved as effective in the treatment of AS as in the treatment of RA. Some – such as gold, D-penicillamine and hydroxychloroquine – are useless. However, sulfasalazine and methotrexate may be helpful in patients with large-joint (extra-spinal) arthritis, and some of the newer agents, such as etanercept, may turn out to be very useful.

Other Drug Approaches
Corticosteroid injections directly into the sacroiliac joints, under X-ray guidance, may help relieve the pain of very active sacroiliac inflammation. Some recent research suggests that intravenous pamidronate (a drug used to treat osteoporosis) may help patients where other drugs have failed.

Physiotherapy
This is (to coin a phrase) the backbone of treatment in anky-losing spondylitis. In many forms of arthritis, physiotherapy plays a supporting role; in AS its role is central. In the acute phase of AS, physio can contribute a lot to pain relief and the restoration of normal spinal and chest movement.

Hydrotherapy in a swimming pool is one of the best ways to achieve this. Once the acute phase is over, the hard part – sticking to a regular exercise program – begins. It's clear that the eventual outcome of spinal movement depends on the patient's commitment to a daily program of exercise to increase flexibility, strength and fitness. The most useful thing the patient can do is link up with a therapist who understands AS. Once the exercise routine is learned, the patient should get a checkup at least once a year. Spine and chest movements can be measured, and if there is deterioration the program can be changed.

Occupational Therapy

OT is not an issue early in the disease, except for advice on appropriate supportive furniture to ensure good sleeping and working posture. If ankylosis has occurred and the spine has become rigid, then the advice of a therapist is more important.

Surgery

Surgery for AS is uncommon. When it's done, it's usually to replace damaged hips with artificial joints. The patient is invariably a young man, and the problem a combination of pain and severely limited hip movement. Short-term outcomes are excellent. Unfortunately, many patients will require further operations in the years to come, as the metal and plastic parts of the artificial hip wear down.

Education

In AS, as in other forms of arthritis, education is very important. Patients must know how to "read" their bodies and must understand their disease. They have to be in charge of their medication schedule, and they have to understand the thinking behind all aspects of treatment, particularly the exercise program. In many countries, particularly Great Britain and Canada, there are excellent national organizations for patients with AS. They provide members with a variety of material (books, pamphlets, videotapes) as well as regular newsletters.

What Is the Long-term Outlook?

For most patients, it's very good. Since 1947, researchers in Toronto have been following a large number of people with ankylosing spondylitis. At the 30-year mark they made the following observations:

- disability developed primarily in the first 10 years, with little worsening in function after that time
- over 90 percent of patients were coping with the demands of normal daily life very well
- pain continued to be a problem for many, but a third were pain-free

Unlike rheumatoid arthritis, there is no significant increase in overall death rates in AS. Patients should expect a normal life span.

Nowadays, with the benefits of NSAIDs and regular exercise known, there should be little disability from the arthritis unless there is hip-joint damage. Those who smoke should quit; the combination of smoking and a chest that doesn't allow full movement may lead to an increase in infections. If eye inflammation occurs and isn't treated, it may cause, over the years, problems with vision. Finally, those who have truly developed a "poker spine" may be more vulnerable to spinal fractures, even with very minor accidents.

The Arthritis of Inflammatory Bowel Disease

When his doctor phoned me about Dennis, I knew I had to see him right away. Dennis was 28, and his problem was his right knee. Four days earlier it had become swollen and painful. I agreed to see him the next afternoon because the problem had many possible causes and the best way to get a handle on it as soon as possible was to get a needle into the knee.

As it turned out, I was none the wiser after the visit. Yes, after I had drawn off a sample of knee fluid and sent it to the lab I knew that the problem wasn't due to an infection, and that it wasn't a crystal arthritis like gout. But I drew a blank everywhere else. No other joints hurt, this had never happened before, he had no symptoms of any kind other than his knee pain and there was nothing in his family history that might suggest an inherited tendency. I put Dennis on an NSAID and arranged for him to come back in 10 days.

It wasn't a week later that I heard from his doctor again. Dennis had been admitted to hospital with severe abdominal pain. My first thought was that the NSAID had precipitated an ulcer, possibly even a perforation of the stomach. I was wrong. The admitting diagnosis was appendicitis, but once the surgeon opened the abdomen he found an inflamed segment of small bowel. Dennis had Crohn's disease. This was the clue I had needed to diagnose his problem: arthritis of inflammatory bowel disease. This is an arthritis that affects about 10 percent of people with either ulcerative colitis or Crohn's disease, the two main types of inflammatory bowel disease.

Ulcerative colitis and Crohn's disease are conditions where the bowel wall becomes inflamed, ulcerated, and/or scarred. These conditions tend to be chronic, waxing and waning over many years. The cause is unknown, but inheritance may be a factor.

Ulcerative colitis, which affects about 1 in 2,000, is a disease of the large bowel (the colon). It most commonly shows up as abdominal cramps with bloody diarrhea. Crohn's disease affects slightly more people, possibly 1 in 1,500, and can affect both the small and large bowel. Its symptoms are similar to those of ulcerative colitis.

The arthritis of inflammatory bowel disease takes two distinct forms, one involving the arm and leg joints, the other the spine. Either one may be associated with either of the two forms of bowel disease. It's possible for a patient to suffer both forms of arthritis.

The peripheral arthritis tends to:

- be the more common of the two
- involve large joints, especially a knee or an ankle
- affect only a few joints (one to six) at a time
- eventually settle down (half do so within six months)
- not cause joint damage

Peripheral arthritis also tends to be an indicator of bowel inflammation, often showing up just before bowel symptoms appear or reappear (as was the case with Dennis), and improving when the bowel inflammation improves (either spontaneously or as a result of medical or surgical treatment).

Spinal arthritis tends to:

- be similar in symptoms and X-ray changes to ankylosing spondylitis
- be present for some time (even years) before bowel symptoms appear
- show up more as X-ray changes (15 percent) than symptoms (5 percent)
- be associated with HLA-B27 in about half the cases

The spinal form does not usually improve with improvement of the bowel disease, unlike peripheral arthritis.

Both forms of arthritis may be associated with episodic eye inflammation (iritis and conjunctivitis), and/or inflammation where ligaments and tendons attach to the bone (enthesitis).

How Is It Treated?

The peripheral arthritis is best treated by controlling, as completely as possible, the inflammatory bowel disease. This may not be easy. In difficult cases, local injections of corticosteroid can be very effective, particularly if the problem is only in a single joint, such as the knee. Sulfasalazine is a second-line drug that also has clear benefit, although it's no miracle cure. Methotrexate seems to help some patients. In a disease that has "ups and downs," however, individual cases prove nothing. Proof requires a carefully constructed clinical trial and none has been done to date.

The spinal arthritis is more of a problem. NSAIDs such as naproxen or even indomethacin can give good results, but may increase bowel irritation, and patients have to be monitored carefully for that complication. Sulfasalazine has also been used, as an addition to or instead of an NSAID, in an attempt to achieve better overall control.

What Is the Long-term Outlook?

For the peripheral arthritis, the outcome is good. Disability and joint deformity are distinctly unusual.

The outcome in the spinal arthritis is similar to the outcome in ankylosing spondylitis.

Reactive Arthritis (Reiter's Syndrome)

I saw Don on the orthopedic surgery ward. He was trussed up in a splint and bandages. He looked like hell. A 28-year-old farmer, he had been admitted the weekend before with the sudden onset of fever, chills and severe right groin pain. At that time, the pain was so bad that he couldn't bend his leg to slide his pants on. Putting weight on the leg was out of the question. An important piece of information came out at that time. Two weeks before, he had gone to his family doctor complaining of burning on urination and a yellowish discharge from his penis. He admitted to being what is euphemistically referred to as "sexually active," and a tentative diagnosis of gonorrhea was made. He was started on penicillin and, although the culture for gonorrhea came back negative, the burning and discharge cleared up.

The orthopedic surgeon, faced with severe pain in a single joint in a patient who had all the hallmarks of an infection, did the logical thing. He took Don to the operating room, opened up the hip joint and put in a drain. He started Don on intravenous antibiotics.

The reason Don looked like hell, and the reason I was asked to see him, was because he then went on to develop two fiery red eyes. "Bloodshot" was an understatement, though Don did not complain of much pain. The big advantage in coming in late in a case like this is that it often makes more sense to a newcomer. Adding up the picture so far, we had evidence of arthritis, of urethritis (the discharge and burning) and of conjunctivitis (the fiery red eyes). I was pretty sure we had a diagnosis here – of reactive arthritis, or Reiter's syndrome – but I went for the icing on the cake, and found it. The roof of Don's mouth showed a large, reddened (and painless) area of ulceration, and the end of his penis, under the foreskin, was raw and inflamed. Finally, he had another feature that I've seen only a couple of times. The line of the hip incision was marked on either side by a weeping, crusting rash. It looked like psoriasis to me.

Hans Reiter, a German army doctor in the First World War, put his name on this syndrome by describing an officer who developed infectious diarrhea and promptly came down with arthritis, conjunctivitis (eye inflammation) and urethritis (inflammation of the urethra, the passage that empties the bladder).

Since then, a number of things have become clear: the condition is a systemic one, affecting more than joints; most, but not all, patients have the inherited factor HLA-B27; and the condition can be a reaction to a number of infections.

Because of this, the term most commonly used today is "reactive arthritis."

Who Gets Reactive Arthritis?

Reactive arthritis tends to strike young adults, most between ages 20 and 40; it's uncommon in the very young or very old. This fact, and the fact that males are three times more often affected than females, has no ready explanation, because the factors that we know are involved don't discriminate by age or sex. The known specific infectious organisms which can "trigger" an attack of reactive arthritis can occur in anyone, as can the genetic inheritance of HLA-B27 which is present in 75 percent of cases. The disease is fairly rare. Some 30 cases per 100,000 people are identified each year.

Only a handful of infections are felt to be triggers. These are, for the most part, organisms that attack the bowel and the genito-urinary tract. Some patients give a history of major symptoms of infection, some have had only mild symptoms and in some there is nothing to suggest an infection at all.

What Are Its Characteristics?

Arthritis
This is usually what brings the patient to the doctor. It is similar in its variety to all the other forms of spondylarthritis. In general, this means that it involves fewer rather than more joints, larger rather than smaller joints, and

---

Signs and Symptoms of Reactive Arthritis (Reiter's Syndrome)

* arthritis
* symptoms of a triggering infection
* symptoms of a generalized illness
* psoriasis-like skin lesions
* mouth and genital ulceration and inflammation
* bowel and genital symptoms
* eye inflammation

Not all of these occur together in the same patient at the same time. Some patients (probably the majority) develop only one or two of the three characteristics that Hans Reiter described: arthritis, conjunctivitis and urethritis. These people are referred to as having "incomplete Reiter's syndrome."

---

lower extremities (hips, knees, ankles) rather than upper extremities.

Swollen toes (dactylitis) and tendinitis or enthesitis are frequent. Back pain tends to come on if the arthritis becomes chronic. Joints are commonly very inflamed – red, hot, swollen and painful.

Symptoms of the "Triggering" Illness

The patient may recall these preceding the arthritis by a week or two. These may include burning with urination, a discharge from the penis, cramps, diarrhea and abdominal pain severe enough to raise concern about appendicitis. In many people such symptoms are so mild as to pass without complaint, and in about 10 percent no symptoms can be recalled.

General Symptoms

Feelings of severe illness are common: fever, sweats, loss of appetite, profound fatigue.

Psoriasis-like Lesions

Eruptions of weeping and scaling skin may develop on the

palms and soles of the feet, or the nails and skin may develop changes that look like typical psoriasis.

Mouth and Genital Ulceration and Inflammation
Shallow, painless, inflamed ulcerations may be seen in the mouth and, in the male, under the foreskin.

Bowel and Genital Symptoms
Urinary burning and penile discharge may develop even when, as in the case of Hans Reiter's Prussian officer, the triggering event was an intestinal infection. The reverse is also true. A genital infection due to chlamydia may provoke abdominal cramps and diarrhea.

Eye Inflammation
Inflammation of one or both eyes is easily spotted and may be the first sign of the reactive arthritis. It has a tendency to recur, and because it can cause serious eye injury with the passage of time it's important that an eye specialist examine the patient. Long-term follow-up may be necessary.

In 1984 the Pope came to Canada, and celebrated a large open-air mass in Ontario. Many police officers from across the province were assigned to the event. Each was given a box lunch which contained, among other things, salmonella bacteria. The food had been contaminated by a salmonella carrier. A total of 1,608 officers were exposed to this unexpected treat, and almost 30 percent developed symptoms of infection.

Since this strain of salmonella is a known cause of reactive arthritis, Dr. Rob Inman and his colleagues in Toronto attempted to contact all who were infected. They sent out questionnaires and followed them up through the officers' family doctors. Of the slightly more than 400 who were infected, 27 (or 6.5 percent) developed reactive arthritis. Nine cleared completely within four months, but at five years the other 18 were still having problems with arthritis.

How Is Reactive Arthritis Treated?
As with the other forms of seronegative spondylarthritis, it's the symptoms that are treated, initially with NSAIDs. Corticosteroids may be necessary, either by mouth or by injection into the joint. Second-line drugs are generally not used. However, if it looks as though the attack is going to be more drawn out, an agent such as sulfasalazine may be used.

Antibiotic treatment is still controversial. One recent research study suggested that antibiotics, given daily over a matter of months, may reduce symptom severity and shorten the period of illness.

The patient should be seen at least once by an eye specialist, because evidence of eye inflammation (though usually obvious) may be subtle and require a very careful examination.

What Is the Long-term Outlook?
For most patients it is excellent. The acute inflammation in the joints usually settles down within weeks to months. But many people will experience some form of recurring symptoms over the years. These may simply be episodes of stiffness and soreness, particularly in the lower back. One patient in three will suffer deterioration of the sacroiliac joints, visible on X-rays. Some will experience ongoing and quite disabling arthritis.

Eye and genital inflammation may have an even greater tendency to recur than the arthritis.

Systemic Lupus Erythematosus (SLE)
Laura is 23 years old and in her second year of medical school. I had met her briefly the previous year as a student in my clinical skills class. At that time I had been struck by the red, scaling rash on her face. It looked very familiar to me. So when she came to me just after Christmas and told me she had lupus I wasn't too surprised. What did surprise me was that she had

made the diagnosis herself. So my job, after I had confirmed that she was right, was to determine how much she knew, what she feared and what she was prepared to accept.

The rash had begun a year before. It was red and splotchy, bumpy in some areas and flat in others, with a tendency to flake. It was on her forehead, her chin and the tip of her nose – but especially on the cheekbones just below her eyes. She had seen a skin specialist and had been given a cortisone cream. This had helped, but as the summer came on and she was outdoors more and more the rash worsened again.

A month before I saw Laura she developed arthritis. Her wrists and fingers were stiff and painful, and there was swelling of many knuckles. Her shoulders, knees and the balls of her feet were also stiff, particularly when she got up in the morning. It took her 45 minutes to loosen up. Her family doctor made an appointment for her to see me, and at her request ordered an ANA (antinuclear antibody) test. He also started her on an NSAID, ibuprofen, and this helped take the edge off the pain.

When I saw her, I learned a bit more. She had been experiencing mild hair loss all year. It wasn't enough to be noticeable to anyone else, but each morning she would notice a dozen strands of hair on her pillow. She had also been feeling very tired, her appetite was poor and over the year she had dropped about 5 pounds below her usual 110. She said she did not have Raynaud's phenomenon (see later), sores in her mouth, dry eyes, pleurisy or other chest pain. She was on no medication but the birth control pill.

Most significantly, her father had been diagnosed as having systemic lupus erythematosus some 20 years earlier. Knowing this, when arthritis developed, Laura went first to the medical sciences library and then to her family doctor. The requested ANA was positive.

I carried out a general physical examination. There were no surprises. Aside from some puffiness of her middle knuckles on all fingers of both hands, and traces of the rash on her cheeks, there wasn't much to find. This was one situation where laboratory testing would be important.

In systemic lupus erythematosus (SLE), also known simply as "lupus," there is inflammation in many parts of the body. The joints are usually affected, which is why these patients come to me, but so are (or can be) many other areas – in particular, the skin, the blood, the kidneys, the nervous system and the tissues lining the heart and lungs.

SLE seems to be a disease of the immune system gone crazy. Antibodies (the proteins normally formed to protect the body against foreign invaders such as bacteria and viruses) appear to be formed against many of an individual's own tissues. These antibodies seem to trigger inflammatory reactions in skin, joints and all the other areas that show up in symptoms.

Who Gets SLE?

Women are 10 times more frequently affected than men, and an onset between ages 15 and 25 is considered typical, though a recent British study put the age of onset squarely in middle age. It's much less common than rheumatoid arthritis; in North America there are possibly four new cases a year for every 100,000 people. In the United States, blacks have it at three times the rate of whites, and there is a slight tendency for more than one member of a family to be affected. Occasionally, drugs (such as procainamide, used for heart rhythm disturbances) can cause it, in men as well as women.

What Are the Characteristics?

Lupus has many faces. A rheumatologist usually sees a case that includes arthritis, a nephrologist sees one that includes

type of symptom	present initially	present eventually
• general	75%	85%
• skin changes	50%	80%
• mouth sores	20%	30%
• arthritis	60%	90%
• pleurisy/pericarditis	20%	50%
• nervous system	25%	50%

lab abnormalities		
• kidney	45%	50%
• blood	15% or less	50%
• antibodies	95%+	95%+

kidney disease, a dermatologist sees one where skin rash is prominent, and so on. As time goes by, a wider range of characteristics tends to develop. But in the individual patient, only one or two of these features may dominate and some patients never go further.

General Symptoms
These aren't unique to lupus, but are indicators that the patient is "all over sick," the state typical of, for instance, many severe infections. Fever is often part of this in lupus, as is a loss of both appetite and weight. But in SLE, possibly more so than in other types of arthritis, the symptom of overwhelming fatigue is striking.

When I first heard about Roger from his family doctor, to say that I didn't accept his diagnosis of lupus would be an understatement. For one thing, Roger is male, and for another thing he is well and truly middle-aged at 49. He also lacks almost all of the general features of lupus. What he does have is the following:

- profound fatigue – this started a year ago. He loved to cycle and play tennis, and he suddenly discovered that he couldn't even climb stairs without stopping on the way up to rest. An effort like mowing the lawn would leave him exhausted for days. He had been forced to take sick leave from his job as a youth counselor six months earlier, and he had come to believe that he would probably be unable to work again.

- profound depression, starting about the same time. It was so bad that he even considered suicide. Fortunately he sought psychiatric help, and his depression, if not cured, was at least improved.

- stiffness and soreness, coming and going, in the knees, hips and buttocks. It occasionally wakened him at night when he turned over, but for the most part it was tolerable.

- loss of appetite and a 10-pound (4.5 kg) weight loss

If I had seen Roger with only that information, I would not have put lupus anywhere near the top of my list. But, fortunately for Roger, he had a psychiatrist who was puzzled by the picture and followed up an astute hunch. He ordered a series of tests. One was the ANA test and the other was the anti-DNA test (see below), and both were positive. The ANA test told me that lupus was possible, and the anti-DNA test indicated that a diagnosis of lupus was inescapable, even if he didn't have all the American College of Rheumatology criteria for lupus.

I put Roger on prednisone, 15 milligrams a day, and I saw him three weeks later. His life had been transformed. He felt wonderful. His energy had returned, he was back at work and he had resumed his tennis game. I outlined a schedule for reducing the prednisone, told him as much about lupus as I felt he could deal with in one sitting and made the first of a long string of follow-up appointments.

Skin Changes

There are a number of ways the skin reacts in lupus. One of the most common – seen in about a third of cases – is the *"butterfly" rash*. This is a reddish, slightly raised rash over the cheekbones (the "wings" of the butterfly) and bridge of the nose. It may be itchy or slightly painful, and is often worsened (or first brought out) by exposure to sunlight.

The *discoid lupus rash* is less spectacular. It consists of bumps or small plaques with thickened scales covering them. These are chronic – that is, they persist for months or years. With time the central area of the plaques may become thin, flattened and white. This rash is common on the face, in the cheekbone area, but can be found in the scalp or in other sun-exposed areas. Many people with discoid lupus don't have systemic lupus, though some may, after many years of skin rash only, develop the systemic form.

The rash of *subacute cutaneous lupus* is halfway between the two already mentioned. Sunlight seems to affect it very much. This is the rash that Laura had. Some doctors feel that this kind of rash indicates a milder form of lupus, but I don't think that's always the case.

Hair loss, or alopecia, is very common – it appears in about a third of cases – and seems to act as a marker of the level of activity. It improves as the patient improves and, as in Laura's case, seems to increase when the lupus flares. Hair loss is almost always diffuse, and not obvious unless carefully looked for. Bald spots are very uncommon.

Photosensitivity is a problem for about half of all patients. Exposure to sunlight causes a skin rash to develop or (as in

Laura's case) get worse. In some cases photosensitivity extends beyond the skin, and can provoke a generalized flare-up of lupus. Because of this risk I tell most of my patients to stay out of the sun. If this is unavoidable, I urge them to wear hats and long sleeves, and to use sunscreen.

Raynaud's phenomenon is a striking series of events that involve the fingers, and sometimes the toes, in up to half of lupus patients (as well as a large number of otherwise healthy people). With exposure to cold, a finger – one, several or all – goes white and loses all feeling. With rewarming the finger (or fingers) becomes bluish or fiery red (or both) and there is an intense burning sensation.

Mouth Sores

Recurring painful ulcerations within the mouth or nose, and sometimes in women in the vaginal area, are fortunately not common. They tend to improve as the lupus improves.

Colleen and I have known each other for a little over 15 years. We first met in the hospital lab, where she works as a technologist. At that time she was 23. Almost immediately she became my patient. Her lupus came on quite suddenly. Initially it was a severe reaction to the sun – her face became beet-red and swollen, and stayed that way for three days. This was followed, over the next several months, by a series of symptoms that raised serious concern. She began to experience drenching night sweats, felt constantly feverish and was exhausted. Mononucleosis was the initial suspect, until her hands and feet became puffy and painful and she developed shallow ulcers on her tongue and the roof of her mouth. That, and the fact that she developed a typical "butterfly" rash on her nose and cheeks, made the diagnosis obvious. The laboratory tests were, as expected, positive for lupus.

Colleen has been on prednisone almost all of the intervening years. For the first several years the daily dose ranged from 20 to 40 milligrams, with occasional bursts up to 60. Every time we attempted to lower the dose to a reasonable level, Colleen would develop more joint pain and new ulcers would appear in her mouth. Most uncomfortably, she also began having similar painful ulcerations in the vaginal area. Her rash and hair loss tended to have parallel flare-ups.

Ten years ago Colleen ruptured her left Achilles tendon. She had a few days warning of pain at the back of her ankle, and then the tendon gave way. It was impossibly painful for her to stand on the toes of her left foot. With an ankle cast she healed, although she is still very weak on that side. The right ankle threatened to repeat the experience five years ago, but it settled down before the tendon actually ruptured. This is a known but very uncommon complication of lupus. Prednisone is also suspected as contributing to the tendon weakness.

The only other area of difficulty has been periodic recurrences of painful bluish discolorations and occasional cracking of the skin at the tips of some of her fingers and toes. These too – which I think are due to inflammation in very small blood vessels – seem to come and go with the other signs of her lupus.

What I haven't seen at any stage, despite careful searching, is any evidence of kidney involvement. Examinations of urine specimens, and blood checks for abnormal kidney functioning, remain consistently normal.

Colleen has done much better in the last few years – ever since I added methotrexate to the prednisone. Methotrexate, a drug that I use a great deal to suppress the inflammation in rheumatoid arthritis, seems to have a similar effect in lupus. It has allowed us to lower Colleen's prednisone to a very low level – less than 5 milligrams a day – without any major return of her joint pains or mouth ulcerations.

Arthritis

This is one of the most common features in lupus. It occurs in the same pattern as rheumatoid arthritis (RA) – involving many joints, small and large, on both sides of the body, and in particular the knuckles of the fingers.

There are a couple of big differences from RA, however. The arthritis tends to be milder, responds to treatment more easily and does *not* result in cartilage and bone damage. While the intense inflammation in the fingers may cause finger deformity, this is quite uncommon (less than 10 percent). When it does happen, it's because of inflammatory weakening of the ligaments supporting the joints.

Joint pains (arthralgia) without obvious inflammation are as common as swollen joints. And, as Colleen demonstrated, tendons (particularly large ones like the Achilles tendon or the tendon that anchors the kneecap to the upper shinbone) may become weakened and even rupture.

Pleurisy/Pericarditis

Inflammation of the covering (the pleura) of the lungs is called pleurisy, and inflammation of the lining of the heart (the pericardium) is called pericarditis. Evidence of inflammation in these two locations is commonly found in lupus patients if it is looked for carefully, but the inflammation itself is usually without symptoms. When symptoms do occur, though, they can be very unpleasant.

The pain of pleurisy is sharp, "like a knife in the side," on one side of the chest or the other, and is made much worse by deep breathing and coughing.

Pericardial pain can be very similar to the pain of a heart attack; it is usually described as "heavy" or "crushing," occurs in the center of the chest and, like heart attack pain, may also spread into the neck or the arm.

Both types of pain usually respond quite quickly to treatment, which is usually prednisone. Sometimes inflammation in these locations is linked to small local collections of fluid in the spaces around the lung or heart, but it is extremely rare for these collections to cause trouble.

Inflammation can also happen within the heart and lung tissues, and in the heart such inflammation can damage the heart valves. When this happens, the damage may cause "heart murmurs" (abnormal sounds detectable by stethoscope). Almost always, however, inflammation in these locations is silent, unsuspected and without serious consequences.

Nervous System

The nervous system includes the brain, the spinal cord and the network of nerves that travel throughout the body. Almost every part of the nervous system can be affected by lupus inflammation. The two most common problems, however, are headache, usually of the migraine type, and difficulties with concentration, memory and learning.

A number of other effects are not common but quite serious and are almost certainly caused by lupus. These include coma, seizures, stroke and nerve damage. Psychiatric symptoms, in particular severe depression, may dominate. In fact, depression appears to be the most common symptom of nervous system lupus.

Sorting out these problems, trying to determine if they are caused by lupus itself, by the treatment of lupus, or by some other factor, is very difficult. However, the more severe consequences often respond to intensive treatment of the lupus.

I was a bit surprised when, on New Year's Day, I was called by a colleague of mine about Mary Anne. I had seen her just three weeks before and she had been doing well. She wasn't now, and my friend had just admitted her to hospital.

Mary Anne was a 43-year-old mother of two and a part-time physiotherapist. I had seen her during her first hospital admission the previous October, when a diagnosis of lupus was made. At that time she had quite a few features of the disease, including joint pain and stiffness, Raynaud's phenomenon, a reddish rash on her face, fever and severe depression. She also had abnormal urine; testing showed both protein and red blood cells. Blood tests showed both a positive ANA and a positive anti-DNA, and a kidney biopsy showed "diffuse proliferative glomerulonephritis" – one of the more severe forms of kidney inflammation. I gave her prednisone in a fairly high dose of 60 milligrams a day, and by the time she went home in mid-November she was considerably better. Just before Christmas I saw her again. She was still very tired, hadn't regained the 10 pounds she had lost, but the joint pains and rash had cleared. I added hydroxychloroquine and outlined a schedule for slowly reducing the prednisone over the next three weeks.

Now she was back, and the picture was quite different. Just about the time I was sitting down for Christmas dinner, Mary Anne developed a headache. It was dull and steady, across the forehead area. She wasn't used to having a headache, and she certainly wasn't ready for this one. It kept getting worse and worse. Headache pills didn't help, and when her family doctor gave her a shot of meperidine (a very strong narcotic) it didn't work either. She began to vomit, and that's when she came to hospital and was admitted to the neurology ward. The next morning she developed double vision, and it was clear from examination that this was due to a problem with the muscular control of her right eye; the sixth cranial nerve wasn't working.

I filled her neurologist in on the background, and together we concluded that the most likely cause of both the headache and the nerve weakness was lupus. Mary Anne was given a series of "pulses" of high-dose cortisone intravenously, and the effect was impressive. Within 24 hours the headache was gone, and by the end of the week her double vision had cleared.

That was 10 years ago. Mary Anne stayed on hydroxychloroquine, and over the next few years she gradually discontinued prednisone entirely. There have been two occasions when I prescribed an NSAID for short periods because of a return of her joint stiffness and soreness. Depression has continued to be troubling, and she has been helped by counseling. But she has had no further evidence of involvement of the central nervous system, and her kidney function has returned to normal.

Kidney Inflammation

Like just about every other part of the body, if the kidneys are carefully studied in patients with lupus, some abnormality will usually be found. And as with just about every part of the body, these abnormalities can be very serious but usually aren't.

Most commonly the abnormality shows up on urinalysis, as microscopic traces of blood, or high levels of protein. Blood can leak into the urine anywhere from the kidney to the bladder and the urethra (the passage from the bladder to the great outdoors). If the routine urine test turns up blood cells, I ask the lab to search the specimen again for "red cell casts." These are microscopic cylinders of red blood cells, and they indicate that the bleeding is coming from the filtering unit in the kidney called the "glomerulus." Inflammation in the glomerulus can also cause the filter to become extra "leaky" – the "holes in the sieve" become larger, and albumin in the blood, normally too large to pass through, gets into the urine. If too much albumin is lost in this way, it usually shows up as edema (fluid retention), with puffiness and swelling – particularly of the ankles and feet.

Tests of kidney function (such as blood tests for creatinine and blood urea nitrogen) are usually normal. Both of these substances are filtered out of the blood by the kidney, and passed into the urine, and if their level in the blood rises it usually means that there has been a significant reduction in kidney function.

In the past, kidney failure was one of the major causes of death in lupus. It still is, but in the last 40 years treatment has made a real difference. But it's very important to be alert to the development of kidney inflammation, since there are no symptoms until the damage has been done. Testing of urine and blood at regular intervals is the best way to reassure everyone that no problems are developing.

There is still debate among doctors as to whether a kidney biopsy should be done in lupus patients who show urine abnormalities. This involves inserting a hollow needle through the skin of the back and into the kidney. A tiny core of tissue is extracted and studied under the microscope. The procedure is usually quite safe, but a very small number of patients require blood transfusions to correct bleeding after their biopsies.

When I was recently asked to see Marsha, it was to renew an acquaintance that goes back 26 years. She was 25 when we first met, and for most of the previous year, starting a month after the birth of her last child, she had been plagued by generalized inflammatory arthritis. She had none of the other features of lupus – no rash, no mouth or vaginal ulcerations, no anemia and no kidney problems. But she told me about one episode that might have been pleurisy. To me her problem looked like rheumatoid arthritis, but testing showed the markers for lupus; there could be no mistake. For the next few years, arthritis was the main issue. I treated her with both prednisone and hydroxy-chloroquine, and she did extremely well. As usual, I adjusted the dose of prednisone to the minimum needed to suppress symptoms.

Then, after eight years, it became apparent that Marsha's problem truly was systemic. She developed more joint and muscle pain, and fever and night sweats. She developed an ulcer inside her nose that wouldn't heal. She became anemic, and this was shown to be due to antibodies against her own red blood cells. Finally, after several months, her urine began to show red blood cells, red cell casts and protein. A kidney biopsy showed generalized inflammation of the kidney – the official report was "diffuse proliferative glomerulonephritis," the same diagnosis given Mary Anne.

I increased the dose of prednisone and added azathioprine, a drug designed to suppress the immune reaction. Marsha responded. The joint and muscle pain vanished, as did her fever, and even the urine abnormalities improved.

I seldom saw Marsha over the next decade. She was followed mostly by her family doctor, although she was also seen periodically by a kidney specialist, and I would get copies of his notes. From them I could see that she required very little in the way of prednisone to control her lupus symptoms. I could also follow, unfortunately, the gradual decline in her kidney function as reflected in her lab tests.

Earlier this year I was asked to see Marsha again. I learned that two years ago her kidney function had deteriorated to the point that she had to begin dialysis. Three times weekly she comes into the hospital for several hours to have a machine do what her kidneys can't. She is still working in the municipal planning office. She has no functional impairment (she needs no help either at home or in the office) and she has had no symptoms of active lupus for over 10 years. This phenomenon is well known since the symptoms of lupus often disappear when significant kidney failure develops. She remains on low-dose prednisone, but we are going to try to slowly eliminate even this.

Looking back on the past 25 years, I often ask myself what I might have done differently. Even now our knowledge regarding preventive treatment of kidney damage is imperfect. I have always been concerned that an aggressive approach, using high-dose prednisone and immune-suppressing drugs, might cause far more harm than it remedied. Within the last ten years or so, some proof has emerged that cyclophosphamide modifies the downhill course. Had we known that at the time, we might have used it on Marsha, and risked some of the problems that drug can cause.

Blood Changes

In the blood, there are three major types of cells:

- red blood cells, or erythrocytes ("erythro-" = red; "-cyte" = cell)
- white blood cells, or leukocytes ("leuko-" = white)
- platelets, or thrombocytes ("thrombo-" = clot)

In lupus, there may be reductions in the numbers of any or all of these.

Anemia, or reduction in red blood cells, is usually not severe but can add to the general level of fatigue. Usually the anemia is low-grade and develops in a manner similar to the anemia in rheumatoid arthritis, as a result of inflammation slowing new blood formation in the bone marrow. Anemia can also result from bleeding in the stomach or bowel because of NSAIDs.

Sometimes, though, the anemia is quite severe and is caused by lupus antibodies directed against the blood cells, resulting in their premature destruction. This is called "autoimmune hemolytic anemia." This process of antibodies attacking the patient's own blood cells can also happen with white blood cells and platelets.

Leukopenia, or reduction in white blood cells, occurs commonly in lupus but is without symptoms. There are more than enough white blood cells to fight infection, though treatment with certain drugs may complicate matters and make infection a real concern.

Thrombocytopenia, or reduction in platelets, is much less common (possibly occurring in about 5 percent of cases) and is usually without symptoms. Because platelets are important in blood clotting, if the reduction is bad enough it may cause easy bruising and even bleeding. This tendency to bruising is the first sign of lupus for some patients. It usually responds quickly to treatment with prednisone.

Hélène has been my patient and friend for 30 years. A native of Paris who teaches French in the primary schools, she first came to me when she was 35. Even then, although it had not been diagnosed, she had had lupus for at least nine years. Her attacks of arthritis gradually became more and more frequent and widespread. Her fingers and wrists, knees, ankles and balls of her feet were variably swollen and tender. Fatigue had developed and, some two years before, Raynaud's phenomenon had appeared.

It was her family doctor who discovered that Hélène was anemic. The condition was quite severe – her blood count was about half what it should have been. Investigations led to the discovery of antibodies directed against her red blood cells, and turned up a positive LE (lupus erythematosus) cell test which was at that time the best test we had for lupus.

I started Hélène on prednisone, and within a month her red cell count had doubled. She also regained 5 of the 10 pounds she had lost. I added chloroquine to her treatment.

Over the years I have continued to see Hélène, although not very often; the intervals are often as long as two years. These visits give me a chance to renew our acquaintance, practice my rusty French and keep an eye on her. We have both learned that the most common expression of her lupus is exhaustion. When it returns, and it does so at least once a year, prednisone is the only effective way to deal with it. She has also had recurring problems with a rash on her face, neck and arms. Now she uses a sunscreen whenever she goes outside in the summer. For a period ten years ago she awakened regularly with a severe cramp in the center of her chest, a cramp that seemed to spread into her neck and left arm. An electrocardiogram and cardiac stress test were both normal, so I was pretty sure this was pericarditis and not coronary heart disease. The fact that her pain settled down with an increased dose of prednisone confirmed this.

Hélène remains on a low dose of prednisone most of the time. If it's stopped completely she invariably runs into difficulty – usually with fatigue. Her anemia and her arthritis have never come back.

Antibodies

The main antibodies tested for in lupus (there are many, many more) are:

- antinuclear antibody (ANA)
- anti-DNA
- anti-ENA
- anticardiolipin (aCL)

These tests are used to help pin down a diagnosis of lupus. Whether they can also be used to look into the future of an individual patient is debatable.

The *antinuclear antibody (ANA)* test is very sensitive but not very specific. In other words, it will be positive in just about everyone with lupus – 95 percent of all patients will be picked up. Unfortunately, so will a lot of other people including those with other forms of arthritis, such as many that might superficially be confused with lupus, and many normal people. About a quarter of all 60-year-olds will have a positive test. So it is used as a "screen" – if it's negative and the patient doesn't have a rash that looks like subacute cutaneous lupus (see above), the doctor stops worrying about lupus. (Patients with subacute cutaneous lupus may be ANA-negative, but they are usually ENA-positive.)

The *anti-DNA* test is just the reverse. This test, which detects antibodies to the genetic material of the cell, is not very sensitive; many patients with lupus will never develop a positive test. However, if the result is positive, the diagnosis is lupus; the test is extremely specific.

The *anti-ENA* test detects antibodies against a number of proteins in the cell nucleus. Some of these are very specific for lupus, while others can be detected in other conditions.

Anticardiolipin antibodies occur in some patients with lupus. Some (not all) people with anticardiolipin antibodies will develop the "antiphospholipid antibody syndrome," which is marked by a tendency to form blood clots. These may show up in a wide variety of ways such as phlebitis (vein inflammation with blood clot development) and a tendency toward fetal death and miscarriage. A few lupus patients experience stroke and other neurological catastrophes, and anti-cardiolipin antibodies may be implicated in these.

It has been known for some time that one of the tests for syphilis (VDRL) was more likely to be positive because of lupus than because of syphilis. In fact, a false-positive VDRL became one of the diagnostic points in favor of lupus. We know now that the antibody responsible for this is an anticardiolipin antibody.

How Is SLE Diagnosed?

Diagnosis is easy if a patient comes into my office with a number of lupus symptoms. Often, though, only one symptom is prominent at the beginning. Since I'm a rheumatologist, what I usually see is joint pain. If the story the patient tells suggests non-joint symptoms – a suspicious skin rash, sensitivity to the sun, severe chest pain, Raynaud's phenomenon – an ANA test is performed, which picks up at least 95 percent of all patients with lupus. An ANA test is done as well if the blood count or the urinalysis raises the suspicion of lupus, and on any young woman with joint pain. A negative result usually indicates that we're not dealing with lupus.

If the ANA test is negative but there are enough symptoms to raise suspicions, the ENA test should be ordered.

If the patient has only a few symptoms – such as joint pain – and the ANA test is positive, a diagnosis of lupus is hard to make. Some patients need to be followed and tested for years before the picture becomes crystal-clear.

How Is SLE Treated?

Lupus is a lifelong disease. As in rheumatoid arthritis, the treatment of SLE involves a long-term partnership between the patient and the rheumatologist. Both need to learn how the individual's unique form of lupus affects that person, and how a variety of influences, including drugs, impact on the disease.

Special attention needs to be paid to factors that might stir up problems – infections, reactions to drugs such as antibiotics, and exposure to the sun. A sunscreen with a protection factor of at least 30 is required if exposure to sunlight is unavoidable. Patients should get an annual flu shot, and those who have had their spleens surgically removed (one form of treatment for a low platelet count) should be vaccinated against pneumococcal infections.

In women, some medications used in lupus may be harmful to a pregnancy, and birth control will be important if these drugs are used. Birth control is also important during flare-ups, as pregnancy is best avoided until the disease settles down. But because estrogens may play a role in lupus, low-estrogen pills are recommended.

If the lupus is active, adequate rest is important – even to the point of taking time off from regular activities.

Regular checkups, both physical and laboratory, are important to monitor lupus activity. This isn't always easy. It may be hard to tell old lupus injury from new injury, particularly in the case of the kidney, and medications may cause side effects that confuse the issue. Blood tests may raise suspicions of a lupus flare, either current or incipient, but by themselves they are unreliable. There really is no substitute for an experienced doctor and a long-term relationship.

The drugs used for lupus are also used for other types of arthritis, and will be discussed in greater detail in a separate chapter. Nevertheless, a few "lupus-specific" points should be covered.

NSAIDs

NSAIDs (nonsteroidal anti-inflammatory drugs) are used in lupus much as they are in rheumatoid arthritis (RA). They can be helpful in suppressing very mild joint symptoms but, as in RA, they often aren't sufficient on their own. However, they may help enough that only low doses of corticosteroids are needed to finish the job. Care must be taken not to combine them with more than 7.5 milligrams a day of prednisone, because the combination creates an increased risk of stomach bleeding.

There are two other concerns about NSAIDs. If there is a degree of kidney damage, NSAIDs may cause kidney function to deteriorate further. And sometimes NSAIDs cause symptoms that can be mistaken for lupus. Ibuprofen, in particular, will sometimes provoke fever, headache, neck stiffness and confusion. When the NSAID is stopped, these symptoms resolve.

Corticosteroids

Corticosteroids, like prednisone, were first used in the treatment of lupus in 1950, and the effect on survival was immediate and dramatic. It's not an overstatement to say that, in lupus, steroids are life-saving.

Fatigue, fever, arthritis and skin rash may respond to fairly low doses of 10 to 15 milligrams of prednisone a day. Nervous system involvement, severe blood abnormalities and active kidney disease may require much higher doses, although more than 60 milligrams a day is probably never indicated. It's a trial-and-error situation. Ideally, all of the drug is taken as a single morning dose, but if the flare-up is particularly severe the dose may have to be divided into two or three, and taken morning, noon and night. After the inflammatory flare-up is under control, the dose is maintained for a week or two and then slowly tapered down. As time goes on, most patients learn what a safe rate is, and how low they can go before a flare-up is inevitable.

For many patients, then, corticosteroids are an unavoidable part of lupus. The side effects and complications of these drugs have to be learned, and distinguished by both the patient and the doctor from the lupus itself. The section on these drugs should be reviewed carefully.

Antimalarials

These drugs, used to prevent and treat malaria, were accidentally found to be helpful in lupus of the skin. Since then they have been used to treat other aspects of lupus, including joint pains, fever and fatigue, as well as the inflammation of rheumatoid and psoriatic arthritis.

Hydroxychloroquine is a particularly safe drug, but its maximum effect may not be felt for several months. It's not a "first-string" agent; its use facilitates less use of other drugs, particularly corticosteroids. If hydroxychloroquine seems to help, it should be continued long-term, even if it appears the lupus is in remission, or the lupus is likely to flare up again.

Investigational Drugs

Drugs which have not been officially approved for use in lupus, despite years of experience, are called "investigational." The main agents in this category are methotrexate, azathioprine and cyclophosphamide. The effect of using methotrexate as another anti-inflammatory should permit a reduction of the dose of prednisone. Cyclophosphamide has been shown to slow the progression of severe kidney inflammation, and delay or eliminate the need for kidney dialysis.

What Is the Long-term Outlook?

Lupus has changed from a disease that caused the death of half of its victims within five years of diagnosis to one where 90 percent survive five years and almost the same number live ten years from diagnosis.

There are many reasons for this change, but undoubtedly the discovery of corticosteroids, and their use in lupus, is the most important. It is likely that these drugs not only suppress symptomatic inflammation – arthritis, skin rash, pleurisy, mouth ulcers – but also reduce the number of patients who develop important kidney complications.

Graph showing improved prognosis in lupus over 40 years.

The first five years are the most important. It's usually during this time that people find out what kind of lupus they have. Serious organ involvement, such as kidney inflammation, seldom develops after the first five years. Deaths that occur during that time tend to be caused by severe and uncontrolled lupus, particularly if the kidneys or brain are affected.

Predictors of a Poor Outcome

- kidney involvement
- nervous system involvement
- high blood cholesterol
- high blood pressure
- need for long-term high-dose drug treatment
- African descent

Lupus is a disease of relatively brief flare-ups separated by long periods of apparent inactivity. The only exception to "what-you-see-is-what-you-get" is kidney involvement, where flare-ups can be quite silent. This underlines the importance of periodic blood and urine testing, over the long term. About 85 percent of patients whose kidneys are unaffected will survive 15 years, but this figure drops to 60 percent if the kidneys are involved.

Severe nervous system involvement is also predictive of a poor outcome. Hypertension, high blood pressure, has been identified as a further factor and/or another reason for careful, long-term monitoring.

Treatment itself is not without risk. Long-term, high-dose prednisone or "investigational drug" treatment may be complicated by a number of problems. Severe infection is one real worry. Similarly, treatment may lead to atherosclerosis (hardening of the arteries) by causing a long-term rise in cholesterol and other fats; there is some evidence that antimalarials counteract this effect.

There may also be racial aspects to survival, even when the effects of socio-economic status are allowed for; in the United States, blacks with lupus have a poorer outcome than whites.

Polymyalgia Rheumatica (PMR)

My father mentioned it in an offhand manner. "I must be getting old," he said, "I can barely make it down the stairs to breakfast." The rheumatologist in me was suddenly awake. Even though I knew I was on thin ice (the jobs of being a doctor and of being a son should be kept separate) I asked Dad to tell me a bit more. Very severe stiffness had been waking him every morning for the past three weeks. He was stiff in the neck, the muscles over the shoulders and down into the upper arms, the buttocks and the thighs. He found it painful to sit up in bed and make his way into the bathroom. He had to inch his way downstairs, gripping the railing tightly for support.

By the time he finished preparing breakfast he could move

much more freely and with less pain. What didn't make sense to him, however, was the fact that when he had finished breakfast and the morning paper he was stiff all over again. It took less time to get loosened up then, but the same pattern was repeated throughout the day; rest would bring on stiffness and activity would improve things.

These symptoms, and the fact that Dad was 73, added up to a diagnosis of polymyalgia rheumatica (PMR). Reversing the usual order, I referred Dad to his family doctor. He listened to the story, examined him, checked his sedimentation rate and reached the same conclusion. Then he started Dad on prednisone, and within days the pain was gone. "I can't believe it! Prednisone is a miracle drug!" The testimonial was familiar, and added to my certainty that PMR was indeed the diagnosis.

That was over ten years ago. Dad is now off prednisone (he was on it for about five years, most of the time on very low doses) and his symptoms have cleared completely. I don't expect them to return.

Polymyalgia rheumatica, loosely translated, means "many muscles hurt with rheumatism."

We still don't know its cause, although heredity may play a role. Because it usually starts so suddenly, with flu-like symptoms, a viral cause has been sought, but none found.

Who gets PMR?

PMR is rare under age 50, but in the over-70s it's more common than rheumatoid arthritis, affecting about 3 in every 100 people. As is so often the case with arthritis, there is a sex difference – women are affected two to three times more often than men. It also seems to be primarily a disease of Caucasians living in the northern hemisphere.

What Are the Characteristics of PMR?

In most cases stiffness comes on suddenly and patients can often recall the day and even the hour it started. Others experience a more gradual onset. Either way, the pattern is typical – symmetrical (involving both sides equally) muscle pain and stiffness in a shoulder and hip girdle ("shawl and shorts") distribution. Symptoms may spread up the back of the neck to the base of the skull, and tenderness of the buttocks after prolonged sitting is typical, but the muscles of the forearms and calves are spared. Sometimes stiffness is more localized, and when that occurs it's usually the shoulder region that hurts. The muscles may seem to be weak, but they aren't; it simply hurts too much to use them.

As in all forms of inflammatory pain, the symptoms grow worse with rest, and may even awaken the person at night. They are most pronounced first thing in the morning, and are made much better by movement.

There may be suggestions of a more general problem – fever and night sweats; loss of appetite, weight and energy.

A few people also have some joint swelling, at the knee or the wrist, most commonly, but it's usually mild and fleeting.

How is PMR Diagnosed?

There is really very little else that looks like PMR. In the typical case, there isn't much question.

Sometimes, especially if the patient has joint swelling, the problem is confused with rheumatoid arthritis. Time and the response to prednisone help settle the issue.

Malignancy can look like PMR, particularly if the cancer involves the bone. A careful examination and a short trial of prednisone are helpful since cancer pain doesn't vanish with prednisone. Low thyroid function and hidden infection are other things to be considered, as well as a bone condition –

Signs and Symptoms of Polymyalgia Rheumatica (PMR)
- muscle stiffness in shoulder and hip girdle
- usually abrupt onset
- symmetrical pattern
- pain with inflammatory characteristics
- fever and fatigue
- occasionally joint swelling and pain
- spectacular response to prednisone
- eventually, disappearance of symptoms

osteomalacia, due to vitamin D deficiency – which can be confused with PMR.

The most consistent laboratory abnormality is a high sedimentation rate, which generally reflects inflammation. In PMR it is usually higher than in other forms of arthritis. The saying in rheumatology circles is "Both the patient and the sed rate are over 50."

But the most definitive feature of PMR is the effectiveness of prednisone. Symptoms literally vanish overnight with even relatively low doses, which would be most unusual for other forms of arthritis.

How Is PMR Treated?

Prednisone is not only diagnostic and therapeutic, it's also just about the only drug that really works. But in view of its possible side effects, it must be used with caution (see the section on corticosteroids, in Chapter 7).

The rule with prednisone in PMR is "Go up suddenly, go down slowly."

What Is the Long-term Outlook?

PMR does eventually go away. In some people this happens within the first six months, on average it takes about three years, and infrequently it may take five years or more. Unfortunately, a few people still need to take 1 or 2 milligrams of prednisone each day to keep symptoms away, even after ten years, and I have had the occasional patient who, after a remission of a year or so, had a repeat attack of PMR.

Controlling PMR with prednisone

"Up fast, down slow": With flareups, the dose of prednisone is increased by the patient. As symptoms subside, the dose is gradually reduced.

The Problem of Giant-cell Arteritis (GCA) and PMR

I had been following Sister Monica, a 76-year-old nun, for a little over a year. Her words, in a note she first brought with her, say it well. "One day in March [two months earlier] I awoke aching from head to toe. . . . The nights were terrific. I was up six to eight times from the pain and got little or no sleep. . . . I'm a bit better now, but still excessively tired and I've gone from 124 to 106 pounds [56 to 48 kg]." Her sedimentation rate was 95 (it's normally less than 20). She was anemic, with a hemoglobin level of 94 (normal at least 125). She fit the profile of PMR perfectly. I started her on low-dose prednisone and she improved dramatically. By July a year later she was taking only 5 milligrams of prednisone and was symptom-free.

Two months later, things weren't going so well. Fatigue and muscle stiffness returned and two weeks before I saw her she developed a "throbbing" tenderness over her temples. Four days later she noticed that her vision was blurred, and a week later she suddenly lost the vision in her left eye.

A biopsy of the left temporal artery (one of the areas that was so tender) showed the microscopic changes of inflammation that are typical of giant-cell arteritis (GCA). She was put back on a higher dose of prednisone. Her headache, stiffness and fatigue cleared promptly. Her left eye vision, unfortunately, did not return.

The case of Sister Monica is an example of something that happens occasionally – a patient with PMR developing another, closely related, condition (in her case, GCA).

Most rheumatologists today consider that PMR and GCA are two ways that the same basic disease expresses itself. Both PMR and GCA occur in the same age group and both exhibit high sedimentation rates and excellent responses to prednisone.

GCA (also known as temporal arteritis), though, is much less common than PMR. It's a condition in which inflammation of blood vessels of the scalp and head may cause:

- severe headache, usually in the temple region (this occurs in about 70 percent with GCA)
- local tenderness, and sometimes redness and swelling, over the inflamed blood vessel
- double vision, blurred vision or partial or total loss of sight (which is permanent)

Although less than 10 percent of those with GCA will experience visual problems, this is the complication that is most feared.

In some patients, such as Sister Monica, the overlap between the two conditions is apparent. Indeed, about half of those with GCA also have the aches and pains of PMR. On the other side of the coin, if a biopsy of the temple artery is done in a patient with PMR (even if there are no scalp symptoms) there is a 10 to 15 percent chance that examination under the microscope will show evidence of GCA.

What, then, is the risk of visual loss for a patient who has only symptoms of PMR? There are no figures, but it's certain that the risk is very low indeed, far lower than the 10 percent risk in GCA.

I've seen only two patients with PMR who suddenly lost vision in one eye. Both were on low doses of prednisone and had no symptoms of either PMR or GCA at the time.

My current practice is to tell my patients with PMR that there is a risk of GCA, that it is extremely small but it can't be eliminated. I tell them that if they ever develop sudden double vision, blurred vision or loss of vision they should take "a handful of prednisone" (twelve 5-milligram tablets) and get to the hospital. Prompt attention may prevent permanent loss of sight in that eye and – even more to be feared – involvement of the other eye. If the second eye does become affected, it almost always occurs within a week of the first.

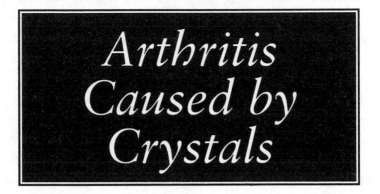

THREE

Arthritis Caused by Crystals

Gout

David, a 42-year-old accountant, spent the weekend in agony. From a vague ache at bedtime Friday night, the pain in his left foot had grown. When he awakened early on Saturday he couldn't bear to have the sheets touch his foot. To stand on it was out of the question, and putting on a shoe was impossible. By the time he hobbled into my office on Monday morning, leaning heavily on a borrowed cane, he hadn't slept for two nights, despite a dozen pain pills. He slipped off a heavy gray wool sock to show me his foot. It was puffy and pink from the instep to the toes. The area surrounding the base of the big toe was cherry-red, swollen, tense and shiny. When I held my hand a half-inch away (he winced in anticipated pain), I could feel the heat.

David had never experienced pain like this before. It was far worse than the fracture he had a month earlier, when his foot got in the way of a hockey puck.

David had no family history of arthritis, and questions revealed no factors that might have provoked this attack of gout. But gout it certainly was. We proved it at his next visit by drawing from the toe joint, through a fine needle, a small drop of bloody fluid that revealed, under the microscope, the bright shiny crystals of the body chemical that causes gout. Before that, however, we had treated David with indomethacin, an NSAID. It took several days before the foot was entirely normal, but by that next visit a week later the swelling, redness and pain had gone.

Gout is the arthritis caused by crystals of sodium urate deposited in the body as a result of long-standing abnormally high levels of uric acid in the blood. In David's case the crystals were in a joint.

Gout crystals also can be deposited in lumps under the skin (known as "tophi") or in the kidney as kidney stones. It is important to keep in mind that gout is curable, and if treatment is started before joint damage occurs the long-term outlook is excellent.

Who Gets Gout?

Gout occurs in people with hyperuricemia – elevated levels of uric acid in the blood. The likelihood of developing gout is directly related to both the degree of excess uric acid and the length of time this abnormality has existed.

Gout is common – in Western societies it affects approximately 2 in every 1,000 people. It's usually a disease of adult men. In the age group from 35 to 45 years, 15 men out of 1,000 will be affected. The number rises with increasing age, but the peak age for the first attack is 50.

Women do get gout, but less frequently – one female for every seven males. The first attack is typically after the age of 60, and in women attacks may involve many joints at once from the beginning.

There is a family history of gout about 20 percent of the time. Gout is also linked to a number of other medical conditions – obesity, hypertension, elevated cholesterol and triglyceride levels, hardening of the arteries and, possibly, diabetes.

What Is Gout Like?

Acute attacks of gout are painful – more painful than almost any other form of arthritis. They come on suddenly, often without warning, sometimes after a few hours of vague discomfort. Single-joint attacks are the rule and any joint may be involved. However, the "bunion" joint at the base of the big toe (the first MTP joint) is the most common. Doctors call this "podagra" (literally, "foot seizure"). After the big toe, the instep, the heel and the ankle are most common sites.

Untreated, attacks last from several days to several weeks. They may be infrequent – once a year or less – especially at the beginning. However, in the vast majority of cases, a second attack follows the first within six months to two years. As time goes by, attacks become more and more frequent – even monthly or weekly. Between attacks, at least in the early years, the affected joints look and feel perfectly normal.

Later on, if treatment of the high uric acid is not begun, about a third of attacks will be *"polyarticular,"* involving a number of joints at the same time. The fever and chills that often accompany this kind of attack can make the doctor worry about the possibility of a blood-borne infection causing *septic* (or *infected*) *arthritis*. This type of attack, though, responds just as well to treatment as the single-joint, *"monarticular"* attack.

Very occasionally, polyarticular gout may be less severe ("subacute"), and so persistent and involving so many joints, both large and small, that it's mistaken for rheumatoid arthritis.

Although not as spectacular, gradual joint deterioration resembling osteoarthritis may develop over time, even in a joint that hasn't been involved in previous acute attacks. It's particularly important for the doctor to be aware of this possibility, because it's entirely preventable with the appropriate use of allopurinol (see below).

How is Gout Diagnosed?

Other kinds of arthritis can be mistaken for gout. Other crystals can cause similar attacks, the commonest being the CPPD crystal of chondrocalcinosis (see next section). Often rheumatoid arthritis will begin with acute attacks of single-joint inflammation, but such attacks are usually less than 72 hours in duration, the big toe is rarely the target and in weeks or months the true problem is gradually revealed.

Finally, whenever any joint becomes suddenly inflamed, particularly if this is the first time, the possibility of a joint infection (septic arthritis) must be considered.

Gout can be diagnosed with absolute certainty only one way – by drawing fluid from a joint ("joint aspiration") and examining it ("synovianalysis") under a polarizing microscope for the tiny crystals of sodium urate. Without such proof, the wrong diagnosis may be made and the wrong treatment started. If the attack is actually due to an infection, the wrong diagnosis may cost the patient the joint, if not his life.

Diagnosing gout from an abnormally high blood level of uric acid is a mistake. The level can be elevated in normal people, especially those taking drugs such as diuretics and ASA in low doses. And many people with acute gout will inexplicably have normal blood levels at that time.

If the patient is a middle-aged man with an acutely swollen big toe, a presumptive diagnosis of gout can certainly be made. But before a lifetime of treatment is prescribed, microscopic proof of the crystals' existence should be obtained.

Two other forms of proof, not as iron-clad as joint aspiration, are sometimes helpful. An X-ray of the foot may show evidence of bone erosion where uric acid deposits have worn away part of the surface of the bone. A 24-hour urine collection may show evidence of excessive uric acid production and excretion, and reveal the small number of patients who are at risk of kidney-stone attacks.

What Causes Gout?

Uric acid is a normal body chemical, the product of a process known as "purine metabolism." It is derived both from the breakdown of protein in food and from the ongoing process of body tissue breakdown and repair. Some is reused by body tissues and some is excreted into the intestine, but most is disposed of by the kidneys.

Uric acid: The cause of gout

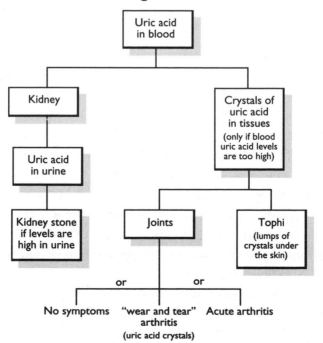

In normal individuals, uric acid levels in the body remain constant because the rate of disposal by way of the kidneys matches the amount added each day through diet and tissue growth. But the process is out of balance in people who are either "underexcretors" or "overproducers."

In underexcretors (the majority of people who have gout) the kidneys filter almost all new uric acid, but a small amount is retained each day and over time more and more accumulates in the body. This has to go on for an average of 20 to 30 years before the first attack of gouty arthritis occurs. During this time, the excess uric acid is deposited in body tissues as crystals of sodium urate, because the blood simply can't carry that much uric acid in a dissolved state. An average person has about one gram of uric acid in the body. In gout the amount is two to four times higher, almost all in crystal form. In joints, crystals take the form of whitish deposits; under the skin, they form lumps or "tophi." Tophi are seldom detectable at the time of the first attack, but about half of all untreated patients will have them after ten years.

This kidney defect is usually inherited, and the kidneys are otherwise normal. However, some medications, particularly diuretics (drugs used to treat high blood pressure and fluid retention) can affect the kidneys the same way. If taken for years, they can cause sodium urate to accumulate, resulting in gout. Chronic obesity can have the same effect – not enough to cause gout, but enough to aggravate the situation if gout already exists. Underexcretion can also be caused by long-standing kidney disease. For example, in the southern United States "saturnine gout" is common. This kidney impairment is a result of chronic lead poisoning caused by drinking moonshine whiskey.

Overproduction of uric acid is a cause of gout in less than 10 percent of cases. Research has shown that, in most of these, an inherited abnormality exists. The normally finely tuned process of uric acid production is out of control, and the rising level of blood uric acid no longer signals the body to stop making more. Most people in this category are otherwise normal, but sometimes excess production is due to abnormal cell growth, as in certain chronic blood disorders. Chronic alcohol overuse, particularly beer drinking, also appears to contribute to overproduction, and may aggravate the situation in someone already predisposed to gout.

Because the amount of uric acid filtered by their kidneys is so large, overproducers are particularly at risk for uric acid kidney stones. An attack of "kidney colic" due to such a stone may be the first sign of gout, occurring before the first attack of arthritis. And stones are not only painful; they can lead to kidney damage. It's important, therefore, to identify those who are at risk. This is done by determining the uric acid concentration in a urine specimen collected over 24 hours – the higher the result, the greater the risk and the more important early treatment is.

Why is gout so uncommon in women? It has to do with the blood's uric acid levels. In males, the level rises about 20 percent at puberty. In women it doesn't; until the menopause, women's levels are consistently lower. Only if there is a major inherited abnormality, usually indicated by a very strong family history of gout, do high uric acid levels, and gouty attacks, occur in women during their childbearing years.

What Brings on a Gout Attack?

The sodium urate deposited in joints appears to be inert most of the time. However, for reasons not yet understood, newly formed crystals sometimes provoke a furious reaction within the joint. White blood cells, entering the joint from the bloodstream, attempt to engulf and digest these tiny crystals, much as they attack bacteria and other foreign materials. Urate crystals are, unfortunately, indigestible, and their chemical nature makes them toxic to the white blood cells. These cells literally explode, releasing their digestive enzymes and other chemicals into the joint and amplifying the inflammatory reaction. At its peak this response may involve hundreds of thousands of white blood cells. The result is a joint that shows all the classic signs of inflammation – swelling, heat, redness and pain.

Although we can describe the attack in cellular and bio-chemical terms, we still have little knowledge of the events that immediately precede it. Nor do we have a convincing explanation for the fact that, even without treatment, the attack eventually stops. We can, however, recognize some common situations in which acute gouty attacks occur. These include:

- episodic excesses of alcohol and rich food
- crash diets
- local joint injury
- hospitalization, especially for surgery or heart attack
- the start of drug treatment to lower blood uric acid levels

Folklore links gout to high living, especially binges of alcohol and food. In this case, the story is true. The breakdown of large amounts of alcohol and protein in the body results in a brief but measurable rise in the normally constant level of blood uric acid. Alcohol in particular seems to be harmful – it not only blocks the kidneys' handling of uric acid, it also temporarily increases its production. (Alcohol does this to everyone, but only those who have accumulated sodium urate deposits will suffer attacks of gout.) It's thought that this "blip" in blood level somehow affects the status quo in the joint, so that new crystals are formed, triggering the inflammatory response.

Crash diets, the metabolic changes associated with surgery, and treatment with drugs that lower uric acid all cause similar "blips," but in the majority of attacks we still have no idea as to the triggering events.

How Is Gout Treated?

In theory we should be able to cure gout. We have extremely effective anti-inflammatory drugs; we also have drugs to lower the body stores of uric acid. In practice, however, the road to a cure can be long and difficult.

It is very important for the gout sufferer to know the purpose of each drug prescribed. They are not all the same. Some are to reduce the risk of an attack, some are to cut short attacks that do occur and some are to reduce the body load of uric acid. Until this high body load of uric acid is eliminated – *and this may take several years* – gout attacks can and do continue.

Treatment of Acute Attacks

Today there are a number of drugs which are very effective in treating gout. Most NSAIDs (except ASA), when used in adequate dosages, work better and faster than older treatments like colchicine, and without severe side effects. Treatment started at the first sign of an attack will end it in a matter of minutes to hours. If there is a delay of days, the attack will persist for days.

The "gold standard" of treatment is indomethacin, usually 50 milligrams every six hours at first, and then tapering off as the attack is controlled. Naproxen, piroxicam and other NSAIDs are alternatives. If taking medication by mouth is impossible, as when an attack occurs after surgery or in the presence of a bleeding ulcer, a corticosteroid ("cortisone") given intravenously, by intramuscular injection or even by direct injection into the joint, is the right choice.

For more on NSAIDs and corticosteroids, particularly regarding side effects and precautions, see Chapter 7.

Prevention of Attacks

Colchicine can be used in low doses, daily, to prevent up to 75 percent of recurring attacks. Aside from nausea, which may force a reduction from two tablets to one each day, there are remarkably few side effects. The only caution has to do with people with reduced kidney function, whose dose should be halved. Toxicity, which is rare, occurs when either too much is taken or a normal dose can't be eliminated from the body. The reaction takes the form of profound weakness, with nerve and muscle damage.

Regular doses of NSAIDs such as naproxen can also reduce the frequency of attacks. Unfortunately, neither colchicine nor an NSAID will do anything to reverse the continuing accumulation of sodium urate in body tissues or reduce the risk of insidious joint damage.

Prevention can also mean avoiding many of the things that provoke attacks, such as excesses of alcohol and food at holidays, and crash diets after.

Lowering of Blood Uric Acid Levels

Reducing the uric acid level in the blood and gradually eliminating the body stores of sodium urate is the only way to "cure" gout.

For many years, the only way to do this was with a diet low in protein. Unfortunately, such a diet was almost impossible to maintain and was only partially effective. Today such diets (termed "low purine diets") are rarely used.

In the 1940s and 1950s, two drugs – probenecid and sulfin-pyrazone – were found to promote excretion of uric acid by the kidney. They are still used today in some situations, such as the development of an allergic reaction to allopurinol. Unfortunately, for people who are at risk for urate kidney stones ("overproducers" and therefore "overexcretors") these drugs increase the risk.

Today allopurinol is considered by most rheumatologists to be the best choice. The drug was developed 25 years ago as an agent to block the body enzyme that converts two other chemicals – xanthine and hypoxanthine – into uric acid. It does this very effectively, and with no new production of uric acid the old sodium urate crystal deposits gradually dissolve into uric acid which is excreted. After several years the risk of further gout attacks diminishes, tophi disappear and the formation of kidney stones is stopped. Xanthine and hypox-anthine do not form crystals in the body and are easily excreted by the kidneys.

Allopurinol treatment should be started when:

- gout attacks are so frequent as to interfere with normal life
- there is evidence that joints are being damaged by gout
- tophi are present
- urate kidney stones have been diagnosed
- a 24-hour urine test has detected a significantly raised level of excreted uric acid

Allopurinol may be used in situations where these criteria don't apply, but where the person simply wants freedom from future attacks. Some physicians begin the drug after a single attack, reasoning that an attack implies significant joint accumulation of crystals and inevitable joint damage. However, it is a lifetime treatment – if the allopurinol is stopped the attacks will resume, often within the year.

In my experience, allopurinol is a very safe drug. There are a few things to know about it, however.

Indigestion is probably the most common side effect, and can be reduced by taking allopurinol with food. If ampicillin, a commonly used antibiotic, is taken at the same time as allopurinol, the risk of a skin rash is increased threefold.

Kidney insufficiency, common in older people, also increases the possibility of side effects on the usual dose of allopurinol. Some of these side effects (which can also happen to people with normal kidneys) can be quite serious, such as inflammation involving both the kidneys and the liver, as well as fever and skin rash. For this reason, allopurinol dosage must be reduced in the presence of kidney impairment.

There is another, more common risk in starting allopurinol. We've seen that anything that causes a sudden rise or fall in blood uric acid levels (remember the effect of a rich meal and a few drinks?) can provoke an attack, and this includes allopurinol. Therefore, allopurinol is initiated with colchicine once or twice daily, with a supply of indomethacin handy just in case. After the system has had a chance to adjust to the new routine (to be safe, many doctors wait up to a year) the colchicine is dropped.

If allopurinol is started while an attack is still going on, it prolongs the attack. The right way to introduce it is to control the attack completely with an NSAID such as indomethacin, and start colchicine, to prevent a recurrence, once things have settled down. Only then should allopurinol be introduced.

Since obesity and chronic alcohol intake, particularly of beer, contribute significantly to the build-up of uric acid in the body, measures to correct both should be taken along with any drug therapy.

Finally, drugs should *not* be used to lower an elevated level of uric acid if the person has had no symptoms of gout. The patient may never develop gout. Treatment may be not only unnecessary, but costly and perhaps harmful. It's better to see if there is a reason for the elevated uric acid level and, if possible, deal with it.

Chondrocalcinosis (Calcium Crystal Disease)

Donna is 65 and looking forward to spending the first years of her retirement pursuing her lifelong passion for bird-watching. I'm seeing her after an urgent phone call from the Emergency Room. She's been devastated by the onset, last night, of pain, swelling and warmth in her right knee. Although she was a bit more active than usual this past weekend, hiking the paths that border our local river, she's positive that the knee wasn't injured. This has never occurred before. Her health has always been excellent. Painkillers have only blunted her discomfort, but she is mainly concerned about the implications of the attack. Will this mean she has to change her lifestyle? Will she be crippled?

My initial assessment is acute monoarthritis. I run through the usual range of possibilities – infection, injury with bleeding into the joint, an unusual presentation of rheumatoid arthritis – but based on probabilities, and on the very sudden and intense nature of the attack, arthritis due to a crystal is high on the list. Gout is always a consideration, and Donna is sufficiently post-menopausal to be afflicted, but the syndrome of "pseudo-gout" seems even more likely.

I aspirate the joint. A #25 needle is thin enough that pain is minimal, and I take the synovial fluid to the lab myself. Under the microscope, the field is crowded with white blood cells – and many contain the telltale crystals of calcium pyrophosphate dihydrate. Back in the office, I review the X-rays taken earlier that day. A thin, milky line outlines the knee cartilages. I reach for my prescription pad.

Chondrocalcinosis (CC) refers to joint cartilage ("chondro-") becoming saturated with crystals of calcium ("-calcinosis"). The calcium crystal in this instance is calcium pyrophosphate dihydrate (CPPD). In the majority of cases, there is no arthritis. But some people with this condition do experience episodes of acute arthritis that are indistinguishable from gout; others develop a picture indistinguishable from osteoarthritis.

Who Gets Calcium Crystal Disease?

The X-ray finding of cartilage calcification is common, but in most cases it means nothing. It's found with increasing frequency with advancing age; one study found it in a quarter of those over 85. It affects women twice as often as men.

On the rare occasion that it's found in someone under 50, it may be linked to an underlying disorder – most often hyperparathyroidism (abnormally high activity of the parathyroid gland) or hemochromatosis (a disease characterized by hugely abnormal iron stores in the body). Chondrocalcinosis can also be inherited.

What Are the Characteristics?

I stopped Jim, a stocky 38-year-old laboratory technologist, in the hospital corridor. He was hopping along, one-legged, with the help of crutches. Ruefully he explained that he had come down hard in a weekend soccer match, twisting his right knee. I pushed the cuff of his trousers up and felt his knee. It was hot, swollen and very, very tender. CC was the furthest thing from my mind when, after some persuasion, he allowed me to aspirate the knee. But instead of being bloody, which I expected, the fluid was yellow and very cloudy. In short order we discovered CPPD crystals, found extensive CC on X-rays of his knees and discovered that Jim's blood and liver iron levels were extremely high. Fortunately this condition, hemochromatosis, hadn't been present long enough to cause liver, pancreas or heart damage. Today Jim is a regular blood donor, which keeps his iron levels down, but his X-rays haven't improved. In fact, over the past 20 years a number of joints – his knees, elbow, ankle – have developed what I would call, if I didn't know the reason for the deterioration, osteoarthritis. Jim no longer plays soccer, but he is still a passionate hiker.

CC is without symptoms in the majority of patients with the X-ray abnormality. Symptomatic CC – the peak decade for symptoms is 65 to 75 – can take two forms.

Acute Attacks

This "pseudo-gout" may be indistinguishable from gout, except that the knee is the most common target; the wrist, elbow, shoulder and ankle follow. Big toe attacks are quite uncommon. The speed of onset is similar, as is the untreated duration, from one to three weeks. Most attacks occur without warning, but local injury or medical or surgical stress may precede them. Extremes of drinking and eating rich foods are not implicated. Involvement of more than one joint at a time is rare. Recurring attacks tend to come in clusters, but attacks themselves are far less frequent than gout attacks.

CC may be suspected as a cause of an acutely swollen joint in an older patient if an X-ray shows evidence of chondrocalcinosis. However, joint infection or even gout are equally valid possibilities. Diagnostic certainty demands that the joint be aspirated and the synovial fluid examined for crystals and bacteria. There are no blood tests to detect the condition.

Chronic Arthritis

Chronic pain due to chondrocalcinosis may be mistakenly

labeled "osteoarthritis" (OA) because of many shared features – the pain and crepitus ("grinding" sensations or sounds) with use, a tendency to involve joints like knees and hips, and the appearance of later X-rays (which, because of advanced deterioration, may no longer show the telltale cartilage calcification). There are no figures on how often the mistake is made, but it is probably very common. CC may be one of the most important causes of OA. Its presence should be suspected when X-ray changes like those of OA are seen in joints that are rarely affected by OA – shoulders, elbows, wrists and the knuckles at the base of the index and long fingers – or when there is prolonged morning stiffness or too much joint warmth and swelling. Such evidence of inflammation can be so impressive that rheumatoid arthritis is diagnosed.

Chronic arthritis due to CC is usually only slowly progressive, so most people cope with it well in the long run. Knees and hips, though, often eventually become so troublesome that surgery is necessary. Overall, however, when compared with patients with osteoarthritis, people with this form of CC do much better indeed.

Chondrocalcinosis in the knee

thigh bone (femur)

calcium deposit

cartilage

shin bone (tibia)

How Does Chondrocalcinosis Come About?

A feature that distinguishes CC from gout is that crystal formation occurs *only* in cartilage. CC pyrophosphate, which is a common product of cell metabolism, seems to come mostly from cartilage cells. Why it combines with calcium to form CPPD is unknown, but there may be different reasons for different patients. In most, the phenomenon is linked to aging. In others, trauma is a factor. For example, CC very often occurs in the remaining cartilage after surgical removal of a torn knee cartilage. The excessive weight load borne by the cartilage that remains seems to be the culprit. In some cases, the chemical environment of the cartilage – high levels of calcium (in hyperparathyroidism) or iron (in hemochromatosis) – somehow favors the formation of CPPD crystals.

As with gout, we don't clearly understand what provokes attacks of pseudo-gout. Shedding of crystals into the joint space from their normally safe location deep in cartilage may be caused by local injury when the attack is linked to definite joint trauma, or to infection inside the joint, but doesn't explain attacks that come on with hospitalization for surgery or heart attack. Once crystals appear in the joint, however, the same sort of reaction found in gout develops in a pseudo-gout attack.

How Is It Treated?

Acute attacks are dealt with much as attacks of true gout are – with NSAIDs such as indomethacin or naproxen, or with corticosteroid injection. The latter is often preferable, especially if an easy-to-inject joint, such as a knee, is the target. Not only does this ensure that a very potent drug is placed in precisely the right place, it avoids the risk of NSAID side effects. NSAID complications, such as fluid retention, worsening of chronic kidney insufficiency, or stomach or duodenal ulcer bleeding, are much more frequent in older patients, the same people who develop CC.

Those with chronic CC arthritis, particularly if there is a major inflammatory component or a tendency to acute attacks, are frequently placed on regular daily doses of an NSAID. In those over 65, drugs that protect against stomach bleeding may be prescribed, and side effects should be even more carefully monitored. Simple painkillers such as acetaminophen are often adequate, and consultation with a physiotherapist is worthwhile.

Asymptomatic patients (those who show X-ray evidence of calcification but don't have pain) do not benefit from treatment. No way has yet been devised to reduce the burden of calcium crystallization. Even where an underlying disorder has been discovered and treated effectively, CC will persist.

The Lost Crystals

In 1679 van Leeuwenhoek, an early developer of the microscope, first identified crystals of sodium urate from a tophus (gout deposit), and in the 19th century Garrod found the same crystals clinging to a thread dipped in fluid from a gouty knee.

These lessons were forgotten, however. It wasn't until 1961 that Dan McCarty and Joe Hollander, using the polarizing microscope in Philadelphia, rediscovered urate crystals in gouty joint effusions. They continued to look, and soon stumbled on the CPPD crystals in fluid from inflamed joints that were initially thought to be gouty. The chemical structure of this new crystal was worked out. Finally, the link was made between these crystals and the X-ray diagnosis of chondrocalcinosis.

Non-Inflammatory Arthritis

Osteoarthritis

Osteoarthritis (OA) is sometimes called "degenerative joint disease" or "osteoarthrosis." It's the most common type of arthritis, yet technically speaking it isn't "arthritis" at all, because "-itis" means inflammation and OA usually has very little to do with inflammation. It isn't even a single disease. The best definition is that osteoarthritis is what happens when joint cartilage fails.

Here are four examples of what we call osteoarthritis, each quite different from the others. The four are chosen because they cover the most common and important varieties. Though OA can be found in any joint, it seems to affect primarily four regions – the knees, hips, hands and spine.

Example #1 – Osteoarthritis of the Knee

Catherine is now 69 years old. She and her husband have run a gift shop in a small summer resort town for the past 30 years. I saw her last nine years ago. The problem was the same then as now – her knees. She really doesn't remember when they first began to bother her but it was at least 15 years ago. She has never had a severe flare-up of pain or swelling. She doesn't recall any injury to her knees, and she has never had arthritis anywhere else. She has always been somewhat overweight, but is not obese.

"My knees still aren't much trouble. I really don't have any pain unless I stand or walk a lot. They don't hurt at night. When I first get up in the morning they're a bit stiff, but they're OK after a few minutes. I do have to be careful going down stairs. They don't feel very steady and I worry that they're going to give way on me. When I go out, I use my cane all the time. I know you told me to start using one after my last visit, but I was too proud for a long time. Canes are for old people. But I started to worry about falling, and now I always use it. I wish I'd done it before. The cane does help with the pain, and I can get about much better.

"I tried taking ibuprofen [an NSAID] but I didn't notice that it made much difference. Now, if my knees ache, I just take a couple of acetaminophen. They do swell some, especially if I do a lot of walking, but I haven't noticed that they're very warm. I guess the reason I wanted to see you again is to find out if there's something else I should be doing."

Catherine is dramatically "knock-kneed"; when she stands, her knees touch and her feet are at least 12 inches (30cm) apart. Her knees aren't fully straightened out, either, which means she has to keep her hips slightly bent to stand straight. I go over her knees as she lies on the examining table. They are slightly swollen, but cool to the touch. The swelling is partly due to an accumulation of fluid inside the knee joint, but some is a result of new bone that has grown up along the outside of the joint as part of the healing process. I bend her knees, each in turn. My left hand, cupping the kneecap, can feel a rough grinding sensation. I can almost see the roughened, deeply pitted surfaces of the cartilage. The knees are about 15 degrees from lying flat on the table, and I can only bend them to just past 90 degrees. I'm pretty sure the X-rays will show that new bone growth is interfering with full movement. With the legs resting as flat as possible on the table, I push on the inside of each knee. I can almost straighten out the "knock-knee" deformity. This means there has been a collapse of the outer half of the knee joint – the "lateral joint compartment" – probably because the cartilage there has disappeared.

Another thing I notice is that her quadriceps muscles (the muscles on the front of the thigh) are much smaller and weaker than they should be. I'm pretty sure they can be strengthened by exercise. That will do a lot to help support and protect the knees, and even slow the wearing-out process. This type of exercise is the single most important thing that Catherine can do to reduce the pain.

We spend the rest of the time talking about whether she should be seeing an orthopedic surgeon. Total knee replacement surgery, with metal-and-plastic artificial knees, has come a long way, and is now an extremely good choice for many people. But here there isn't a strong argument for surgery; pain isn't a big problem, and her lifestyle is not significantly curtailed. She would do far better with a referral to a good physiotherapist, who could provide:

- a regular quadriceps-strengthening program
- a program of leg stretching
- instruction in protection of the joint
- assessment and advice regarding footwear
- advice on a fitness program that avoids abusing the knees

Then, if and when pain or disability reaches the point where surgery is appropriate, she'll get a better result.

Osteoarthritis of the knee is one of the most common forms of OA. It occurs in about 10 percent of all people over 65, and in about 2 percent of all adults.

Catherine is typical in many respects. She is a woman, and she is in the older age group. Aside from her being somewhat overweight (a risk factor for knee OA), there are no obvious reasons why her knees should be affected. She has surprisingly little pain despite the appearance of her knees, and has been coping for a long time without a lot of medication. The slow pace of her knee OA is typical. Several studies have shown that when knee X-rays are repeated after 10 years, only about a third show any important worsening.

Catherine is not so typical in that her knee OA involves mostly the lateral compartment (outer half), giving her "knock-knees." This happens in about a quarter of all patients with knee OA. Other parts of the knee are more commonly affected: the medial compartment (inner half) and the patellofemoral space (between the kneecap or patella and the end of the thighbone or femur). Some have OA in more than one compartment of the knee. When the inner half of the knee is affected, the resulting deformity is a "bow-leg." When OA occurs behind the kneecap (patellofemoral OA) there is often much more muscle weakness, pain and disability than with the other kinds. Whichever compartment is involved, the process is usually symmetrical, so you don't see a "knock-knee" on one side and a "bow-leg" on the other.

Another type of patient develops knee OA. These patients are much younger, male and have had some sort of knee injury, and often knee surgery.

Ian fits all of these criteria – he's 28, and four years ago he suffered a triple knee injury in a ski accident. He had arthroscopic surgery to trim the torn cartilage and replace the ligament with "plastic rope." Chances are high that over the next 10 to 20 years he's going to start having knee pain and instability, and some typical X-ray changes.

Here is another example of osteoarthritis, one that is quite different.

Example #2 – Nodal Osteoarthritis of the Hands

Alice is 45. She runs a small business, selling quilting supplies and giving lessons in quilt-making. She's worried. Her hands, which she considers her livelihood, have been giving her increasing difficulty over the past two years. The problem started soon after menopause.

"I don't know what I'll do if I become crippled," she tells me. "I have a cousin with rheumatoid arthritis. Her fingers are so twisted that she can barely hold a cup of tea without using both hands. Is there anything I can do so that doesn't happen to me?"

I look at her hands, and in particular at the knuckles – the MCP joints at the base of each finger, the middle PIP joints, and the end (DIP) joints. The MCP joints look normal to me, but four of the DIPs on each hand, and the index finger PIP joint on her right hand, are enlarged and lumpy. Several of the DIP joints look red as well.

"I didn't pay much attention at first. It started in my right index finger, at the end. It got very swollen, red, and if I banged it, it hurt. I kept hoping it would go away, and after a couple of months it did. But it left the knuckle stiff and bumpy. Then it spread to another knuckle, and the same thing happened. Now two more have started. They ache constantly, and sting if I hit them, and my fingers are all getting stiff. In the morning it takes about 20 minutes to get them loosened up. I've been taking coated ASA, and that helps some."

I ask a few more questions. She is right-handed, and the problem seems to be worse in that hand. She has no symptoms of arthritis except in the hands, and she's in excellent health. She has been asking other members of her family if they've had arthritis. Her mother and two of her three sisters also have "bumpy" knuckles, but none of them has ever noticed redness or much besides some stiffness in the morning.

Alice has nodal osteoarthritis, probably the most common form of OA, affecting about 75 percent of women and 50 percent of men by age 70. In middle age women are affected four times more often than men, and there seems to be an inherited aspect to it. Someone who has it probably has a mother or sisters with it, although inheritance doesn't predict whether it's going to be mild or severe. In women it often comes on at, or just after, the menopause, suggesting a hormonal aspect. Activity also seems to play a role. In right-handed people, more right-hand knuckles are affected, especially in the fingers that are most used.

Many will show local inflammation when the swelling first develops. Redness and marked tenderness usually settle down after several months, leaving the knuckles characteristically "lumpy." Individual knuckles are affected at different times. It's not really possible to predict which one will be involved next, or which will be spared. Eventually no new joints are involved, and the hands remain stable thereafter.

The "lumpiness" is due to new bone being laid down at the margins of the joint. When this lumpiness affects the end (DIP) joints, we speak of Heberden's nodes. (William Heberden was an 18th-century physician who was the first person to pay attention to these "little knobs" – he was also the first person to describe the chest pain we now know as "angina." A Frenchman, Bouchard, took second place – he got his name on the middle [PIP] knobs.) Sometimes, when Heberden's nodes are forming, a small cyst over the knuckle develops. If this is punctured, a clear jelly-like material drains out.

Only very rarely are the MCP joints involved, and when they are, there may be another kind of arthritis in addition to OA.

OA may also occur in the joint at the base of the thumb, where it pivots on the wrist (the thumb CMC, or carpometacarpal, joint. This isn't clearly linked to either DIP or knee OA, and it tends to be worse in the non-dominant hand (on the left in a right-handed person). Pain in this joint may be a real problem, especially when the thumb is needed for pinching. A local cortisone injection may help, and sometimes I ask the occupational therapist to fashion a splint to stabilize this joint. Occasionally, I ask a hand surgeon to assess whether surgery would improve the pain and function.

Nodal OA may be quite uncomfortable at times (and without symptoms at others). It may make the fingers look bent, and may make tight gripping difficult. It does not, however, cause the kind of disability that is associated with finger involvement in other kinds of arthritis.

Finger osteoarthritis

Heberden's node (new bone growth of DIP joint)

Soft tissue swelling

PIP joint

The commonest form of hand arthritis.

We know that people with nodal OA, like those with life-long obesity, are more likely to have OA of the knees. However, they do not get arthritis elsewhere with any greater frequency than might be expected by chance. Also, like OA in general, nodal OA is not part of a systemic disease that affects organs such as the heart, lungs and kidneys.

Example #3 – Osteoarthritis of the Hip

George is a 65-year-old farmer. He still gets up every morning and is out to the barn before breakfast. His son, though, has taken over most of the running of the farm. That's a pretty good thing, because George's right leg has been bothering him more and more over the past two years. His wife, Mary, comes with him to my office. That turns out to be very helpful, because it's obvious that George tries to play down his problem. She isn't about to let him get away with it, not after waiting so long for this appointment.

"It's my right leg, Doc," he says. "I think it's my knee. It's a little stiff when I get out of bed in the morning." Mary chips in, "Sometimes he can't even get his sock and shoe on, and I have to do it for him." "It's OK as long as I don't push it, but if I'm on my feet much I notice it. The aching does make it hard to get to sleep."

I'm a little suspicious since I've been misled before by patients complaining about knee pain when the problem was really in the hip. I ask a few more questions, and I'm glad I did. His pain is mostly in his thigh, in the front of the leg just above the knee. It's in the knee too. But he also mentions that, if he tries to get into the back seat of his son's car, he gets a pain in the right groin that just about takes his breath away.

His wife confirms that he's never been sick a day in his life. She's certain that neither he nor any other family member has ever had arthritis problems.

My examination confirms my suspicion. The right knee is perfectly normal, but he can barely bend the right hip to 90 degrees, can't roll it inward and can't take it out to the side more than 30 degrees. I'll be very surprised if the X-ray doesn't show that the cartilage is completely gone on the right hip joint.

I tell George and Mary that I'd like to do an X-ray. I also want to make an appointment for him to see an orthopedic surgeon. I'm not sure he's ready for surgery right now (in fact, I'm pretty sure he's not), but it will be about four months before he can be seen and the first date for elective surgery probably won't be for a year. There's a very good chance he'll be ready by then. Surgery, with replacement of the joint by an artificial one, is almost certain to make a huge difference in his pain and disability. I tell him this, but I also want him to hear it from the surgeon, who also has to tell him about some of the risks involved.

In the meantime, I'm going to arrange for a physiotherapist to see him, show him how to use a cane properly and give him a muscle-strengthening program.

George has osteoarthritis of the hip. The hip joint is frequently the only one involved in this kind of OA. It's seen about equally in men and women. In a very few cases there's an obvious cause, such as a birth abnormality. Congenital dislocation of the hip is one: an abnormally shallow acetabulum (the cup in the pelvis where the thighbone fits) allows the hip joint to dislocate and cause damage. Another birth abnormality, one leg being longer than the other, can also be a cause.

Hip OA can occur at any age, but most of the patients are in their 60s and 70s. Some cases are like knee OA, and go on for a long time with minor symptoms before surgery is necessary. A very few, probably less than 5 percent, seem to heal on their own. But once most patients are in enough pain to come to see me, they will be more than ready for surgery within two to three years. I usually let the patient define "ready." Pain and disability are a far better guide than the X-ray.

George also demonstrates something doctors call "referred pain." He feels most of his pain in the thigh and knee area, and not where it belongs – in the groin. Most of the time a patient comes to me complaining of hip pain, he or she has pain on the outside of the upper thigh or in the buttock. While pain in these areas may be associated with hip problems, it's usually caused by something else.

Example #4 – Osteoarthritis of the Spine

Sam is 48 and teaches English. He's a good friend, and so didn't hesitate to call me to give him some information and advice. A week ago he awoke with neck pain that ran down as far as his right shoulder. Now, any attempt to turn his head intensifies it, which makes just about anything he does very difficult. Pain pills help a little, but he's starting to worry that he's taking too many. His family doctor arranged X-rays of his neck. Sam was dismayed to learn that the report was "extensive degenerative changes involving most of the facet joints, with narrowing of the intervertebral foramina. There is narrowing of C5-6 and 6-7 disc spaces with significant anterior osteophytes at these levels. Advanced osteoarthritis of the cervical spine." This sounds serious. Sam wants a translation into something he can understand.

I examine him. There is no suggestion that any of the nerves, emerging between the neck vertebrae, are being pressed upon. His reflexes, his strength and his sensation in both arms are all normal. I look at his X-rays. They don't look like the X-rays of a newborn babe, but for someone almost 50 they look pretty good. I have no quarrel with the report, but I know two things Sam doesn't. Almost everybody over 40 has changes like this, some better and some worse; and there is absolutely no telling from the X-ray whether the patient has, or will ever have, neck pain.

So I reassure Sam that he will settle down soon. I refer him to a physiotherapist who will probably see him every day until things improve, each time packing his neck in ice and following that with some gentle traction. She'll give him a soft neck collar to wear to bed at night, and offer some advice about pillows. She will not – and I would not – suggest he see a chiropractor since I would worry that neck manipulation might cause serious nerve and blood-vessel damage.

Sam has spinal osteoarthritis. Spinal OA is so common that it's difficult to consider it a disease. Rather, like gray hair, it's something to be expected as we age. The discs between the vertebrae lose some of their water content, shrink and become less bouncy. We lose an inch in height. The facet joints at the back of the vertebrae, which stabilize the spine while still allowing movement, are pushed together. New bone grows in the places where mechanical stresses are high. Most of the time we aren't even aware this has gone on. Sometimes, however, there is local irritation; we experience pain, the supporting muscles go into spasm to keep movement to a minimum, we get more pain and then we call the doctor. Only very rarely is there a serious problem such as nerve pressure, and even more rarely is surgery indicated.

These changes can be seen anywhere in the spine. They are most commonly associated with symptoms in the back (see the section "Low Back Pain") and, to a lesser extent, in the neck.

So What Is Osteoarthritis?
Osteoarthritis is defined by the changes that are seen on an X-ray of the joint with symptoms. Compared to a normal joint, the X-ray more or less shows, depending on the joint and on how long the problem has been going on:

- narrowing of the space between the bones on each side of the joint (the narrowing occurs because cartilage, which doesn't show up on X-ray, has been worn down);
- thickening of the bone ends on each side of the joint (bone reacts this way because it has lost the protective "cap" of cartilage);
- development of cysts in the bone ends (the thicker new bone isn't as elastic as normal bone, and when weight is put on it, tiny fractures occur. Fluid from the joint, under pressure, works its way through the cracks into the low-pressure bone, where it expands into cysts);
- growth of bone "spurs" at the edges of the joint (this is also the body's attempt at healing and strengthening the damaged joint. The Heberden's nodes of nodal OA are really bone spurs of this type).

By this definition, OA can be found in virtually everyone over 50, and in many much younger people. These changes – I cannot emphasize this too strongly – cause symptoms or problems in very few of the people who have them.

Normal versus osteoarthritic synovial Joint

normal, thick, smooth articular cartilage

regular normal bone texture

smooth joint margin

normal, single cell layered synovium

thin, even capsule

irregular thickening of bone

thickening of the joint capsule

modest inflammation of the joint lining

breakdown of the articular cartilage

bone growth at joint margin

bone cyst

Some changes in the joint don't show up on X-ray:

- the cartilage is cracked with tiny fissures, or pitted with ulcerations
- the lining of the joint is thickened and may be mildly inflamed
- the capsule that surrounds the joint has become thickened
- the fluid that lubricates the joint has increased in volume, is often more watery and contains debris from deteriorating cartilage and some inflammatory white blood cells

These changes will occur in any joint once the cartilage deteriorates. All four common types of osteoarthritis have really only one thing in common – the cartilage has deteriorated.

How Cartilage Deteriorates

Cartilage is a tough, spongy, whitish layer that covers bone ends where they meet in a joint. It's living tissue that grows, breaks down, and repairs itself. The first step in the development of osteoarthritis occurs when the repair process no longer matches the rate of breakdown. Sometimes this happens because the cartilage itself is abnormal, such as in chondrocalcinosis. In most cases, though, cartilage breakdown occurs because abnormal stresses, either mechanical or chemical, are brought to bear on normal cartilage.

Who Gets Osteoarthritis?

At one time, OA was simply thought of as a disease of old age. We know better now. While it's true that the number of people with OA increases with increasing age, many people – even in their 80s – have perfectly normal hips, knees and hands. And we see examples of OA in young and middle-aged adults,

A Brief Lesson on Cartilage

Cartilage has no blood supply and no nerves; it gets its nutrition and oxygen from joint fluid. Its only cells are chondrocytes, which make the cartilage that surrounds them.

Cartilage consists of two main materials: collagen and proteoglycans (PGs). The collagen forms a tight "mesh" of tough cables that anchor the whole cartilage structure to the underlying bone. This mesh traps molecules of proteoglycan. Proteoglycans have two very curious properties – they attract water molecules and, like similar poles of two magnets, repel other proteoglycan molecules. Since they sop up as many water molecules as they can, while repelling all other PG molecules trapped in the collagen mesh, about 80 percent of cartilage is trapped water.

This results in a structure much like one of those "bubbles" that cover tennis courts in the winter. The collagen mesh is the fabric of the bubble, and trapped water molecules are the air that is constantly being blown in.

If you can imagine bouncing up and down on a tennis bubble, you can imagine what happens when you take a step. The cartilage covering the bone ends in the knee (hip, ankle, etc.) is compressed as body-weight pressure squeezes some of the trapped water out onto the surface of the cartilage. This does two things. It provides a thin film of liquid for the two cartilage surfaces to slip and glide on as they move against each other. It also squeezes out waste products, including carbon dioxide, from the cartilage. When the body weight is shifted back to the other leg, the cartilage springs back to its original shape and water is sucked back in by the PGs along with oxygen and nutrients like glucose. So cartilage doesn't need blood vessels for nutrition and oxygen, and to get rid of wastes, as long as it's exercised regularly.

without any obvious reason. This has stimulated research into cartilage, in an attempt to determine if many of these people are born with, or develop, cartilage abnormalities that make them more susceptible to deterioration. We also know that knee OA is more likely in people who have (or have a history of) nodal OA.

The Treatment of Osteoarthritis

There is no single way to treat osteoarthritis. Age and activity level, the joint or joints involved, the nature of symptoms

– all these have to be considered and the picture can change with time. That's why it's important to keep in touch with a knowledgeable doctor.

Once the diagnosis has been made, it's important for the patient to get the message that OA is not simply a disease of "getting old," that things will not inevitably go downhill and that there's a great deal that he or she can do. Occupational therapists and physiotherapists are often the best source of this message, and should be turned to at least as often as the doctor if things aren't going well.

Prevention
There is now strong evidence of significant risk factors for OA of the knees. It is strong enough that attempting to reduce these risks make sense:

- obesity in young women (but not men) is a strong predictor for later knee OA. Those who successfully lose weight (one study suggested as little as 12 pounds or 5.4 kg was important) can reduce their risk by over 50 percent.
- jobs involving climbing more than 10 flights of stairs daily, or repeated kneeling, increase the risk of knee OA threefold and jobs involving repeated squatting increase the risk more than sixfold.
- recreational knee injuries that result in cartilage tears or serious ligament strains increase the risk of knee OA at least threefold.

Repeated attempts to link jogging to later hip or knee OA have failed; in fact, there are now good studies demonstrating the reverse. One American study followed 450 middle-aged runners for 12 years, and found they had fewer joint symptoms, disabilities and medical problems in general than members of a similar group who did not jog regularly. The study continued to follow them a further eight years, into their 60s, and the gap widened. The runners had a third the disabilities of those who didn't jog regularly. However, the same cannot be said for athletes at the elite or professional level – even in non-contact sports such as track and field.

Physiotherapy (PT)

Patients with OA are significantly less fit generally, but aerobic conditioning can change that, and benefits are not limited to the patient's general condition. Restoring fitness in patients with knee OA, by something as simple as supervised indoor walking, has been shown to improve both function and pain significantly. At the same time, the need for medication is reduced.

Localized therapeutic exercise is also a potent weapon in dealing with OA, particularly of the knee and hip. Muscles weakened by lack of use are strengthened, and these provide support and protection to the joints, which are vulnerable to further injury in the course of normal daily activities. Pain is reduced. In addition, attention to the hip and knee, including posture correction, can reduce the likelihood of back pain due to awkward standing and walking.

An experienced physiotherapist (PT) can analyze the problem and prescribe the right exercise routine, and then reassess the problem at a later date, making any necessary adjustments. Physiotherapy can also help to restore a normal range of movement, which is often lost when a joint becomes painful and is used sparingly. There are many settings for therapeutic exercise: a swimming pool, with the water at a comfortable temperature, is a good place to start. Ice packs or hot packs may help somewhat in reducing discomfort, but there is little benefit from most of the electrically powered gadgets that are often used (TENS or transcutaneous nerve stimulation and acupuncture also fit into this category of doubtful treatments). Not least of all, a good physiotherapist can help the patient have a realistic perspective on the problem.

Once learned, the exercise program must be continued daily. This requires commitment; the motivation and the effort must come from the patient. Skipping sessions inevitably results in poor outcome.

Occupational Therapy (OT)

Occupational therapists (OTs) deal with practicalities. They are skilled in assessing the effect of home and workplace activities on the problem, and vice versa. They can then suggest different ways of doing the job, or tools that will make it easier. Something as simple as having a toilet seat raised higher can make a huge difference to a patient with knee OA. A cane, fitted correctly and used properly, can reduce the load on the hip by as much as 30 percent.

OTs are also specialists in providing lightweight splints to support injured joints. Their ability to analyze footwear needs, and to modify shoes with lifts and insole supports, is particularly helpful in OA of the knee, hip and back. For example, placing a soft wedge support into each shoe, under the inner side of the foot, might make a great difference to our "knock-kneed" first patient, Catherine. The popularity of "walking shoes" these days makes the job easier. These provide excellent support and cushioning, at a reasonable price, and can easily be modified for the individual patient.

Drug Therapy

No drug has been shown to reverse or halt the disease process in OA, but drugs can help relieve symptoms.

For many years now, doctors have tended to rely on NSAIDs as first-line treatment of OA. Examples include ASA, ibuprofen, ketoprofen and indomethacin. Although these drugs reduce inflammation and to some extent reduce pain, the results have been at best disappointing, and at worst disastrous. Most people with symptoms from OA are over 60, the age group most likely to have adverse effects from NSAIDs. Worsening of pre-existing kidney and heart conditions is common. Ulcers of the stomach or bowel often strike without warning.

Not only do NSAIDs not protect the joint from further damage, but there's some evidence that the reverse may be true. Indomethacin seems to accelerate hip OA deterioration, and the same may be true with other drugs.

In a very few patients, especially those with nodal OA of the hands, inflammation can be part of the problem. These patients are given a short trial of NSAIDs, particularly if symptoms are significant. If there is no major improvement, or if evidence of side effects appears, the drug is stopped. If a patient says that the NSAIDs helped a lot, risks are discussed and using a drug for "ulcer-protection" is considered, especially if there are any risk factors (see "NSAIDs" in Chapter 7).

Analgesics (painkillers) are probably the most reasonable class of drug to use for OA. For mild to moderate pain, the analgesic of choice is acetaminophen. It can be taken as needed, particularly at the end of the day, when the joint is really aching, or regularly, if pain is constant. But one problem with acetaminophen is that it can make control of blood thinning with warfarin difficult. People on warfarin (Coumadin) – which is commonly used in heart disease – should probably stay away from acetaminophen.

Acetaminophen with codeine can be used if plain acetaminophen doesn't work, but if much is required, or even stronger painkillers are needed, surgery should be considered.

Cortisone-like drugs (such as prednisone), when taken by mouth, have no place in the treatment of OA. If there's a significant amount of inflammation in an OA joint, I sometimes inject it with a long-acting form of cortisone – particularly for OA at the base of the thumb, and to a lesser extent in the knee. If relief is not significant, lasting for weeks to months, the treatment probably shouldn't be repeated. In OA of the knuckles, injections may actually damage the joint, and should be avoided.

A *variety of other approaches*, depending on the particular form of OA, may be tried. In knee OA, injections of a substance called *hylan* or *hyaluronan* may result in substantial relief of pain. The treatment is expensive – a series of injections into a single knee costs several hundred dollars, and it may improve the pain for only six months, if it helps at all. I consider it as a step just before recommending surgery. It certainly is not a substitute for exercise, good footwear and weight loss.

Many of my patients are taking *glucosamine*, often in combination with *chondroitin*, on the theory that this chemical provides the raw material to build new joint cartilage. Some are convinced it helps, others aren't so sure. There has been surprisingly little good research, but what exists does seem to say that these compounds are safe, and they may help with the pain of OA. I encourage my patients to give them at least a three-month trial.

Similarly, research into the use of *hydroxychloroquine* (a drug used in the treatment of RA and SLE) has hinted that it may be helpful in the pain of nodal OA, though whether it retards the development of the bony bumps is an open question.

A number of drugs are applied as creams or lotions over painful joints. The theory is that they are absorbed through the skin and work their way into the region of the damaged joint. I don't have much experience with this, but from what I read these may have a limited role in helping deal with local OA pain. Many contain NSAIDs, and this way of using them does avoid the risks of taking them by mouth.

Another drug, capsaicin, a derivative of chili peppers, may be helpful when applied locally, if nodal or knee OA is very painful. Capsaicin is absorbed through the skin and depletes the nerve ends of "substance P." Substance P is a chemical pain messenger, and if it's not in the nerve endings, pain sensation is reduced. Capsaicin has to be applied several times a day, however, which is a disadvantage. Nevertheless, a recent well-designed study showed that a four-times-daily application of capsaicin did make a difference in pain control.

In the future, expect to hear of drugs that retard cartilage breakdown and promote cartilage repair. These may influence outcome profoundly by acting before deterioration becomes obvious on X-ray.

Surgery

Pain, especially night pain, is the main reason for considering surgery; a significant loss of function is the other. Because surgery can fail, at the time or later, it should never be done unless both patient and surgeon are convinced of its necessity. However, delaying too long may jeopardize the outcome. A patient who hasn't walked for two years because of knee OA is not likely to walk again, ever, even with new metal and plastic knees.

There are a number of surgical possibilities, and these vary with the joint involved.

The *arthroscope*, a small-diameter flexible tube that can penetrate the skin and enter a joint, contains both an optical system for inspecting the joint and the tools needed for microsurgery. It's especially useful in joints that are more painful than the X-ray suggests they should be, not only to size up the problem, but to carry out small repairs. We have also found, through using the arthroscope, that flushing out a joint with a salt solution may give long-lasting relief, so "joint lavage" is becoming another treatment tool, at least in knee OA.

Tibial osteotomy involves cutting into, "breaking" and resetting the shinbone (tibia) in cases of knee OA where the surgeon wants to postpone putting in a new artificial joint. This is sometimes done in younger people who have OA of only one side, or compartment, of the knee. By "bending" the tibia in the right direction, weight can be shifted from the "sick" side of the knee to the normal side.

Joint fusion, operating to fix the joint in one position permanently, is seldom a good choice in large joints such as knees and hips. It may, however, be an excellent choice in patients with severe wrist or elbow pain, or where an important joint, such as a thumb MCP, is unstable.

Total hip arthroplasty is now almost always successful, and total knee replacement is not far behind. There are still failures, almost always after some time – metal and plastic can break down, cement and bone can give way – but patients should expect at least 10 to 15 years before such problems arise. Complications such as infection and phlebitis (postoperative blood clotting in leg veins) are still major concerns. Arthroplasty is done only after serious consideration of the alternatives.

Total arthroplasty for other joints remains in the developmental stage; shoulders and elbows are done occasionally, but usually only for severe pain and then with the knowledge that function may be no better. The next few years will likely bring new materials and new surgical techniques that will result in the same gratifying results as those we see in hips and knees.

Low Back Pain

Dave is 50 and an advertising agency executive. He is addicted to running. There are few mornings when he doesn't get in at least an hour, and some days he "doubles" at noon as well. Six months ago, he put in a long run – a little over two hours – on a Sunday morning. The next day, he became aware of a stiffness across the small of his back. Several hours later he felt sharp pain in that area when he bent over. For the next two weeks he was in misery. Any attempt at forward bending, such as to tie up his shoes, set off a painful spasm. Sleep was safe unless he was on his stomach; then, if he tried to roll over, he would awaken with muscle spasms. He gamely tried to keep running, but it was just too painful. After ten days of rest, the pain was still there, but better. At this point, frustrated, he went to see a chiropractor. X-rays showed narrowing of the disc spaces between the lowest three vertebrae in his back. This, it was explained, required adjustment three times weekly. By the second treatment, Dave's pain was significantly better, and in a week he was back to his usual routine. The chiropractor advised monthly manipulation, indefinitely, to prevent a recurrence, but Dave didn't have the time. He was too busy running. He seems to be cured of his pain.

Acute low back pain is a symptom, not a disease.

The lower back is referred to by doctors as the lumbar spine, or the lumbosacral region. Pain there can arise from many sources. It can come from vertebral bone, from the joints or the intervertebral discs that allow one vertebra to move on another, from the ligaments and muscles that tie them together, from the nerves that emerge from the spinal cord or from the spinal cord itself. Pain can also come from nearby structures, particularly those at the back of the abdomen (pancreas, kidney, gut, large blood vessels).

The spine

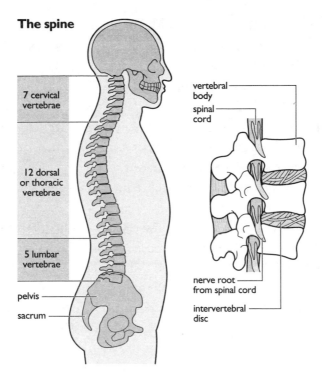

7 cervical vertebrae

12 dorsal or thoracic vertebrae

5 lumbar vertebrae

pelvis

sacrum

vertebral body

spinal cord

nerve root from spinal cord

intervertebral disc

By far the most common back pain is the one Dave experienced. Attempts to pinpoint the source of this type of pain have been failures. Doctors assume it comes from some localized area of injury in the spine. In most cases it's briefly painful and then heals. This type of pain is often spoken of as "mechanical low back pain" to distinguish it from inflammatory back pain. It may be sharp or dull, persistent or intermittent. It's felt in the "hollow" of the back – at waist level, just above the buttocks – but may also spread into one or both buttocks, and occasionally into the back of the thigh.

Pain can develop suddenly, or come on gradually over several days. It may be provoked by an innocent movement, such as bending over, twisting or lifting. It may have no apparent cause. Certain movements may make it quite severe –

forward bending, or arching backward. Coughing, sneezing or other straining movements may make it worse, as may prolonged sitting in an automobile. Rest usually helps a lot.

Some generalizations can be made:

- low back pain is common (in any year 10 to 15 percent of adults will have an attack)
- most low back pain gets better
- the cause of most low back pain is unknown

A sudden attack of low back pain severe enough to interfere with daily life will be experienced, sooner or later, by 80 percent of us. And having had one attack, a third will have another within the following three years. People with back pain make up half of all patients who go to family doctors with "arthritis."

The likelihood of back pain increases with age, but most patients are men in their 30s, 40s and 50s. A job that involves repeated bending, lifting and twisting often seems to be the cause, although a desk job doesn't provide immunity. Bouncing and vibration, as on a tractor seat or the seat of a long-distance truck, are also risk factors. Obesity and smoking seem to increase the risk as well.

Low back pain attacks get better spontaneously. Half are gone within one week, and almost all within eight weeks, no matter what is done; a cynic might say this is why chiropractic manipulation seems to be so helpful. Unfortunately, 5 to 10 percent of cases persist longer than two months. These patients become very frustrated with their pain, and give low back pain its bad reputation. The case of Antonio, described below, is a good example: all too often, patients like Antonio are repeatedly, fruitlessly and expensively investigated. If they are really unlucky, they are also subjected to surgery in a vain attempt at a cure.

The truth is that we can't explain most episodes of back pain. There are many potential causes and a large number of possible sources, but attempts to direct treatment to specific back structures generally end in failure. I think most back pain comes from non-bony tissues, including the muscles that support and protect the spinal column.

Despite this, each new back-pain patient I see requires a careful history and examination. I must make sure that the symptom is indeed the common, garden variety of mechanical low back pain (like Dave's), and not back pain that we can, and must, do something about.

Joanne is 34, an associate professor in the faculty of social science and a mother of two very active preschoolers. Her back pain began like Dave's, with a gradual onset of deep, aching discomfort across the hollow low in the back. Unlike Dave, however, she experienced more and more pain with each day. Soon the pain was constant. Sitting, particularly in an automobile, resulted in terrible intensification of pain; lying in bed required careful positioning with pillows. Sleep was constantly interrupted. After a week, sudden movement, coughing and the straining associated with bowel movements (the pain pills she was taking had given her severe constipation) caused pain to shoot down her right leg and into her foot. The outside of her right foot became numb. I saw her after this had been going on for three weeks. I attempted to raise her right leg from the examining table but at 30 degrees the pain, quickly moving up the leg to her back, prevented going any further. I asked her to stand on one foot and raise her heel clear of the floor. She could do this on the left foot, but not on the right. She was numb on the outer third of the top of her foot. When I struck the back of her ankle with my reflex hammer the usual reaction of calf muscle contraction just didn't happen.

All this – the numbness, the weakness, the loss of the ankle reflex – added up to pressure on a nerve root, and from my examination I was pretty sure this was coming from the very lowest spinal disc space. X-rays of the back were normal, but CT scanning confirmed my suspicion – a protrusion of the disc was causing direct pressure on the nerve root. Here, the clear-cut physical examination findings exactly matched the CT image. Occasions when back surgery can actually be helpful are uncommon, but this was one of them. Joanne had her surgery and today, three years later, the only evidence that she ever had a problem is the continued absence of the ankle reflex.

Acute low back pain with nerve root pressure is uncommon (it occurs in only about 1 percent of people with low back pain), but when it happens, and the pain seems to shoot below the knee in one or both legs, it is called "sciatica." This type of pain is usually sharper, and is often made worse by straining movements. It can be associated with tingling, numbness and even weakness in the lower leg and foot. Sometimes the patient loses control over bladder or bowel emptying (this is very rare, but it's a surgical emergency).

Joanne's case illustrates the importance of a careful physical examination. If testing raises the possibility that there may be pressure on a nerve, further studies – nowadays CT or MRI scanning – are usually done. If the suspicion is confirmed, surgery is usually recommended.

Antonio is 49, and had been an automobile plant production-line supervisor. He hadn't worked for two years, however, and was sent to me for a second opinion. Nine years earlier he'd begun experiencing episodes of intermittent low back pain. These always cleared up in a matter of weeks. Two years ago he again developed pain in the small of his back, which radiated down the back of his upper left thigh. Unfortunately, this time it failed to get better. Indomethacin hadn't helped, and physiotherapy, in his case mostly local application of heat and ultrasound, did nothing. The pain was considerably better when he lay flat, so he spent many hours each day stretched out on the rug at home. Sitting longer than 30 minutes was intolerable, and standing more than 15 minutes had the same effect. He denied feeling numbness and tingling in his legs.

Examination showed a stocky and slightly overweight middle-aged man who moved very gingerly. While sitting, he constantly shifted his weight from buttock to buttock. When I asked him to stand and bend forward he did so, slowly, but was unable to arch backward in the standing position. His muscle strength was excellent. He could walk easily on his heels and his toes. The sensation and reflexes in his legs were normal. Plain X-rays of his back showed some minor narrowing of the L4-5 intervertebral space.

Subsequently Antonio was instructed in a program of flexion exercises, and purchased a portable back support. He has unfortunately not returned to work and is on long-term disability, with no material change in his symptoms.

Chronic low back pain, long-term and persisting despite all interventions, represents only a small fraction of back pain, but constitutes the central problem of back pain in society today. It consumes enormous resources. In 1990 it was estimated that chronic low back pain cost the United States economy, directly or indirectly, almost $30 billion.

We have very little insight into the causes of this problem. Investigations, even such special ones as MRI and CT scanning, can't distinguish these patients from those with episodic back pain or even from many who have never had any trouble with their backs. Anti-inflammatory drugs aren't helpful, and surgery invariably either does nothing or makes things worse.

There are a few things we have learned about patients like Antonio. The longer they are off work, the less likely they are ever to return. After two years, the chances are less than 5 percent.

Recovery from work-related low back pain

The probability of never returning to work increases with time off work after the injury. Adapted from Frymoyer & Cats-Baril (1991).

Edith is 74, a retired librarian who lives with her Labrador retriever in a small country cottage five miles from town. She looks much younger than her years, and hasn't an extra ounce of fat on her body, in part because of her daily rambles across the fields and through the woodlot at the back of her property. In the past six months, however, her walking has been severely curtailed by right buttock and leg discomfort. She describes it as a cross between pain and weakness. It disappears when she's sitting or lying, but comes on with walking. Initially present only on long walks, it has become increasingly easily provoked. Now, just about the time she makes it to the end of the lane to her mailbox, the pain has built to such a pitch that she must sit down. Ten minutes later she can walk again, but she barely makes it home. The same thing happens when she stands to wash dishes at the sink. She has discovered she can make it around the supermarket by leaning forward with both arms on the shopping cart.

My examination turns up very little except that she has limited spinal movement and her ankle reflexes can't be detected (something very common in older people). I can easily feel the blood vessels pulse at her ankles and on the tops of her feet.

Edith has lumbar spinal stenosis – a narrowing of the spinal canal most commonly caused by a combination of backward bulging of the disc, bony overgrowth due to osteoarthritis and thickening of one of the spinal ligaments. The narrowing is aggravated by upright posture, which causes a slight degree of extension (backward bending) in the lower spine, which narrows the spinal dimensions even more. (Leaning forward on the shopping cart tends to flatten out the lumbar spine and "open up" the spinal canal.) Symptoms of spinal stenosis – leg and calf pain with walking – can be mistaken for "intermittent claudication." This is a very similar, and common, pain syndrome caused by narrowing of one or more large arteries in the legs. Her normal foot pulses and the abnormal CT scan of her lower spine helped make up my mind. Like so many other tests, the CT scan is only useful if it confirms the history and physical findings; up to 25 percent of normal people show spinal narrowing on a CT scan but never have a symptom of spinal stenosis.

Many people with spinal stenosis put up with the limitations imposed by the pain and weakness, and some show definite improvement with time. Physiotherapy to strengthen the abdominal muscles and improve spinal posture can help. But some patients, and Edith is one of them, are unwilling to accept their status quo. Edith chose surgery to open up the spinal canal, although she was aware that about a quarter of those who choose surgery end up unhappy with the result.

What Else Can Cause Back Pain?

Inflammation of the Back

This is nowhere as common as mechanical low back pain. For this reason it's often overlooked – which it shouldn't be because, like inflammatory pain elsewhere, it has a characteristic pattern. More important, it can be treated.

It's worse with rest, and often awakens the patient at night. Back stiffness is particularly bad on first arising, and gets much better with physical activity. In contrast, mechanical back pain is almost always better with bed rest and worsens with activity.

The most common type of inflammatory back pain is ankylosing spondylitis. Closely related is the spinal involvement in seronegative arthritis. Back pain may also be part of the picture in polymyalgia rheumatica in older patients. All of these have been covered elsewhere in this book.

Nerve Root and Spinal Cord Pressure

These are usually signaled by sciatica. Pain is not only felt in the low back region, it spills over into the leg, extends below the knee and may be felt as far as the foot. As in the case of Joanne, the most common cause is a bulging (herniated) intervertebral disc. However, there may be more sinister causes. Cancer involving the spine, benign tumors of the spinal canal or infectious abscesses of the spinal canal are all possible causes. Severe, unrelenting back pain that is continuous both day and night is often the clue to one of these.

Problems in the Spinal Column Itself

These include those just mentioned: cancer and infection of either the body of a vertebra or the disc between the vertebrae. The most common cause, however, is a fracture of a vertebral body, and this is almost always due to osteoporosis.

Osteoporosis is the process where bone simply loses its bulk. Bone calcium and the scaffolding on which it's laid down become eroded. When looked at under the microscope, the bone looks moth-eaten instead of being thick and solid.

The typical patient is a post-menopausal woman. Without warning, she develops sudden severe pain in her spine, anywhere from just below the shoulder blades to the lower back. It hurts to move, to cough, to do anything but be very still. Narcotics may be necessary. An X-ray usually confirms the fracture (the vertebral body looks squashed down from its usual square shape into a wedge). The patient gets better, but slowly. By the end of two to three months the pain is gone, but the woman may be just a little bit shorter than she was before.

Pain Referred to the Back from Elsewhere

Such pain, usually from within the abdomen, isn't terribly common. Disease of the pancreas, the stomach and duodenum, the kidneys, and the main abdominal artery (the aorta) can all appear as pain in the back.

How Should Back Pain Be Investigated?

The most important part of the investigation of low back pain is a careful history and physical examination. It's only when things don't make sense, or don't behave as they should, that more is needed. Then the problem is what to choose.

A complete blood count (CBC) and sedimentation rate, two simple blood tests, may be very helpful, especially if inflammation, infection or cancer is on the list of possibilities.

X-rays of the back are almost always a waste of money. Well over half the population over the age of 50 have what appear to be arthritic changes on X-ray. And if these X-rays are mixed up with normal-looking X-rays and a radiologist is asked to judge which patient has back pain, the answer will be wrong half of the time. In fact, many radiologists add to the problem by reporting back to the family doctor, in excruciating detail, every single abnormality, using such words as "severe," "extensive" and "advanced degenerative change." The patient interprets such a report – often incorrectly – as implying severe and potentially disabling damage. However, X-rays may be very useful if there's a question of cancer, fracture, infection or inflammation. I will also ask for them if the pain has been present for a month in spite of treatment.

Other ways to look at the back include CT (or CAT – computerized axial tomography) scanning, MRI (magnetic resonance imaging) or radionuclide bone scanning. They are all, in their individual ways, better at "seeing" spinal structures than plain X-rays. They are also much more expensive and much less freely available. I order them only if I feel that the patient's back pain is different, particularly if I'm considering one of the more unusual causes, or if I'm thinking that surgery may be required.

A note of caution, however. A study reported in *The New England Journal of Medicine* examined MRI testing in almost 100 people with no symptoms of back pain. Half of these patients showed "disc bulging" and a quarter showed "disc herniation." That normal people have "abnormal" results of this nature has been suspected for a long time. Similar findings have arisen from studies of CT scans. The lesson is clear: abnormalities found by CT or MRI testing are only important if they fit the patient's symptoms and findings on examination. To operate on the basis of the imaging test alone is to ensure a failure of surgery.

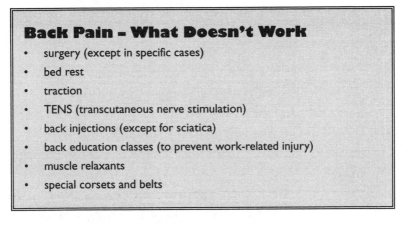

Back Pain – What Doesn't Work

- surgery (except in specific cases)
- bed rest
- traction
- TENS (transcutaneous nerve stimulation)
- back injections (except for sciatica)
- back education classes (to prevent work-related injury)
- muscle relaxants
- special corsets and belts

How Should Back Pain Be Treated?

Obviously the answer varies with the cause, but here I intend to focus on mechanical low back pain of recent onset. Traditionally, treatment has been a choice between the surgical option and the "conservative" option.

The Surgical Option

Back in the late 1930s, Drs. Mixter and Barr popularized the idea that low back pain was caused by herniation (bulging due to weakening of the outer fibers) of the intervertebral disc. As a result, for 40 years patients with low back pain were operated upon, often repeatedly, in an attempt to reduce the disc herniation or to fuse the vertebrae together, or both. Only in the last decade have we come to realize how ineffective and harmful this usually was. Those few people with clear-cut nerve pressure were helped enormously. But many others, those whose pain we still can't explain, experienced only continued, if not worsened, pain and disability.

If there is definite nerve root pressure, surgical relief of that pressure is usually extremely helpful. But even in these cases, surgery is not always the only way to improvement. I have had patients who refused surgery and got better. Since MRI studies have shown that disc bulges often resolve on their own, this is not surprising.

My current practice is to recommend surgery only if:

- the patient's symptoms and my examination point to nerve pressure, *and*
- the CT or MRI agrees with my findings, *and*
- the pain continues to be disabling despite the passage of time,

or

- I find evidence that nerve damage is getting worse

or

- the patient has symptoms of loss of bladder or bowel control.

The "Conservative" Option

Bed rest, usually for at least two weeks, was the rule 25 years ago, but now we recommend either no rest in bed or rest for only a brief period – preferably just a day or two, until the acute pain passes. Then we try to get the patient moving again. But a number of more specific treatments are also available.

Various *back injections* have been used. The most effective involves injecting the lumbar epidural space (the space between the covering of the spinal cord and the bone of the spinal canal) with a mixture of corticosteroid and long-acting local anesthetic. This is done to relieve very severe pain, particularly if there is sciatica. It may be necessary to repeat injections over several weeks, but the relief provided can be considerable.

Anti-inflammatory drugs and painkillers may be very useful, particularly in pain of recent onset. They may allow the patient to resume normal activity more quickly. Since there is generally little or no inflammation in the usual type of back pain, anti-inflammatories, if they do help, usually do so because they also have painkilling properties. Some doctors also prescribe muscle relaxants, but they have never been proved effective.

Various appliances are also available – from the infrared, ultrasound, shortwave diathermy and interferential machines in physiotherapy departments, to corsets and back braces, and the more recent portable TENS (transcutaneous electrical nerve stimulation) units. The best that can be said of these is that they do no harm – the worst that their use wastes a great deal of time and money. They should never be used, as they are too often, as the sole treatment.

Chiropractic manipulation may be worth a try, at least if the back pain is of recent onset and is not going away. A British study comparing chiropractic and traditional physiotherapy for *recent-onset* back pain found that patients treated by chiropractors felt better faster.

An American study compared the outcomes of acute low back pain patients treated by family doctors, orthopedic surgeons and chiropractors. There was no difference in outcome – recovery of function was rapid in almost all patients – but chiropractic treatment was associated with both higher costs and greater patient satisfaction with the treatment.

Current Recommendations for Treatment of Acute Low Back Pain

Since virtually all acute back pain will settle down without any treatment, most experts in the field now recommend that people in the early stages – three to four weeks – be given whatever is needed for pain, reassured of the high probability of complete recovery and strongly urged to get back to work as quickly as possible. If early return to work full-time is just too difficult, a return on a part-time basis should be sought.

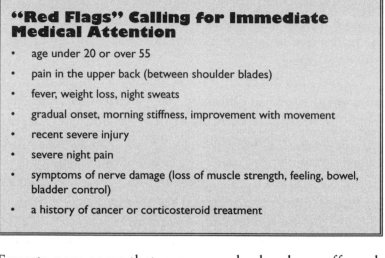

"Red Flags" Calling for Immediate Medical Attention

- age under 20 or over 55
- pain in the upper back (between shoulder blades)
- fever, weight loss, night sweats
- gradual onset, morning stiffness, improvement with movement
- recent severe injury
- severe night pain
- symptoms of nerve damage (loss of muscle strength, feeling, bowel, bladder control)
- a history of cancer or corticosteroid treatment

Experts now agree that someone who has been off work between four and twelve weeks is an entirely different problem. He or she is in real danger of long-term difficulties, as measured by a successful return to work.

A first step is a reassessment by the doctor to check for an uncommon, potentially treatable condition (see box). Then the principles of "intensive work-related case management" are applied. Absolutely essential is the cooperative collaboration of the worker and the employer, often with the assistance of a physiotherapist and occupational therapist. The focus is on the job. The specific activity involved is analyzed. The specifics of the job may be modified, or the hours on that task reduced, or the worker may be involved in a specific work-hardening exercise program – or a combination of all three. (A work-hardening exercise program gradually adapts the worker to the physical demands of the job.) In workplaces where programs such as these are available, time lost from work in the first year may be reduced by up to 50 percent.

Rules for a Healthy Back

- become aerobically fit, and keep it up

- get rid of belly fat

- learn a simple routine of back strengthening and flexibility exercise, and do it

- adopt good work postures, especially for lifting

- wear comfortable, supportive, cushioned, low-heeled work shoes

---

Fibromyalgia (Fibrositis)

Mary Jane is a 40-year-old woman who balances managing a household and three active teenagers with her full-time job in the medical records department of our hospital. She looks tired and very worried. I ask her why she has come to see me. Her answer is one I've heard so many times before; I have to remind myself that jumping to conclusions is not an official Olympic event.

"Doctor, I hurt all over."

I ask her to be more specific, and it soon becomes obvious that her pain is indeed widespread – in her neck, her arms, her back and her legs. It's also clear that she points as much to the muscles as to the joints.

"It's been going on for at least six months. At first I thought it was the flu – everyone else in the family had it – but even after the fever and headache cleared up, my muscles still ached."

By now I can almost predict her answers to my next questions.

"Am I tired? I wake up tired. I feel so weak some days I don't believe I'm going to make it to bedtime. And I'm not getting a good night's sleep. The littlest thing seems to wake me up, and my husband says I'm tossing and turning all night. And I'm so stiff in the morning! It takes me hours to get loose."

Mary Jane has a number of other symptoms I've come to recognize as typical. She has always had problems with migraine, but lately the headaches have become much more frequent. She has developed symptoms of irritable bowel syndrome – morning clusters of crampy lower abdominal pain ending in, and temporarily relieved by, a loose, watery bowel movement. She has tried taking a variety of anti-inflammatory medications, but they don't work. The worst thing, she says, is that she looks so well. None of her joints are swollen, and her family is beginning to think her problem is in her head.

I examine her – first a quick general physical examination to make sure there is nothing else, and then a more specific assessment, looking for tenderness at each of the nine pairs of fibromyalgia tender points. As I go over each of these, pressing firmly with my thumb, she pulls away in obvious discomfort. She seems amazed that I know exactly where to touch to bring out her pain.

Fibromyalgia is a syndrome defined by widespread musculoskeletal pain for at least three months, and abnormal tenderness to pressure on at least 11 of 18 specific points.

In order to meet the definition, pain has to be on both right and left sides of the body, and above and below the waist. The tenderness can be measured by pressing each point with an instrument called a "dolorimeter" (literally, "pain meter"). Most commonly, though, each location is checked by firm thumb pressure. A number of nearby "control" sites are also pressed to make sure the "tender points" are truly not normal.

Who Gets Fibromyalgia?

While the typical patient is a middle-aged woman, slightly overweight and relatively physically unfit, there are a lot of exceptions. I see teenagers and the elderly, along with the athletic, with fibromyalgia. It is one of the most common diagnoses I make.

Chronic pain, felt throughout the body, is common. Studies in both Britain and the United States have come up with similar figures – about 11 percent of the adult population "hurts all over."

The much more specific form of generalized pain, what we call fibromyalgia, is also common, though less so. Probably the best and most meticulously carried out investigation was one done in Canada. It showed that, in a large urban center, almost 6 percent of women and 2 percent of men met the definition. This makes fibromyalgia almost four times as common as rheumatoid arthritis.

The tender points in fibromyalgia

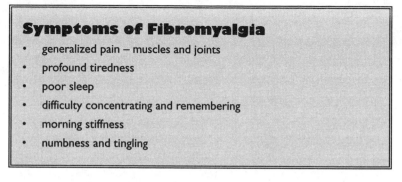

Symptoms of Fibromyalgia

- generalized pain – muscles and joints
- profound tiredness
- poor sleep
- difficulty concentrating and remembering
- morning stiffness
- numbness and tingling

What Are the Characteristics of Fibromyalgia?

Muscle Pain

This is variously described as aching, gnawing or burning, and is the hallmark of fibromyalgia. Mary Jane had difficulty in telling me where, precisely, she hurt; the best she could do was indicate "all over." In contrast, my examination pinpointed a large number of locations where she was extremely tender, and before I did so, she was unaware of any of them. When I pressed firmly over other nearby areas, and over her joints, I couldn't get the same reaction.

Fatigue

This is often so severe that the patient believes there's something wrong with the muscle, but the results of extensive muscle testing are always normal, and strength is actually quite good. However, the combination of pain and fatigue is deadly. The quality of life has been studied in patients with fibromyalgia, and has been found to be as poor as in patients with chronic obstructive lung disease and insulin-dependent diabetes.

Disturbed Sleep

This might be better described as restless sleep, with a tendency to waken easily. This feature may give a clue as to the cause, at least in some people. Drs. Hugh Smythe and Harvey Moldofsky, working in Toronto in the 1970s, discovered that patients with fibromyalgia don't sleep the way normal people do. Sleep patterns can be traced on an EEG (electroencephalogram). Normal people range up and down, from very light sleep (Stage I) to very deep sleep (Stage IV), many times throughout the night. People with fibromyalgia do this as well, but their Stage IV sleep (also called "slow wave" or restorative sleep) is "contaminated" with Stage I sleep, as if they never quite fully relax. Smythe and Moldofsky did something very interesting: they took normal volunteers and hooked them up to EEG machines in the sleep lab, and whenever the volunteers entered Stage IV sleep they were roused slightly – not enough to wake them, but enough to disturb their EEG tracings. After several nights of this, the volunteers started waking up tired, stiff and hurting all over.

Morning Stiffness

This is one exception to the rule that this symptom is an indicator of inflammation. Testing never detects evidence of inflammation, and symptoms do not respond to treatment for inflammation unless (see below) the fibromyalgia is associated with another type of arthritis. Because morning stiffness is so often combined with fatigue, patients often describe awakening as if they "had been run over by a truck."

Other Symptoms

Patients often tell me of numbness and tingling in their hands, though there is never evidence of nerve irritation. They commonly mention that their hands and fingers feel swollen, though there's no swelling that I can detect. Headache and bowel irritability occur in about 50 percent of cases, and current or past depression and anxiety attacks in about 25 percent – more often than would be expected by chance. It's not clear whether there's a cause-and-effect relationship with the fibromyalgic pain. What is clear is that many people with chronic pain become depressed and anxious, particularly if their doctors can't find anything wrong. They suspect the worst, and when a name can be put to their problem they're delighted.

Look-alikes

Superficially, at least, fibromyalgia may be mistaken for one of any number of rheumatic disorders, including systemic lupus erythematosus, polymyositis (an inflammatory disorder of muscle), polymyalgia rheumatica and even rheumatoid arthritis.

Hypothyroidism (abnormally low function of the thyroid gland) is a diagnosis I've been fooled on, though, so I make it a habit to order a TSH (Thyroid Stimulating Hormone) test on everyone who gets a label of "fibromyalgia." Unlike fibromyalgia, hypothyroidism is easy, and very satisfying, to treat.

All of these look-alikes have characteristic findings on physical examination, and they usually show definite abnormalities on lab testing. This is quite different from fibromyalgia, where the usual lab tests are normal.

What Causes Fibromyalgia?

No one knows. Despite its name ("myalgia" means muscle pain and "fibro-" refers to the tissue surrounding muscle fibers), no specific abnormalities of muscle have been found.

There may be many causes.

Trauma, either physical or emotional, is suspected in some cases, simply because of the timing. Some patients' symptoms follow automobile accidents. Some investigators have also raised the possibility of "microtrauma" as a factor in at least perpetuating the disease. They point out that most patients with fibromyalgia are generally out of shape, and their muscles are more susceptible to small injuries in normal everyday use.

Infection is often suspected as a cause. Commonly, as in Mary Jane's case, the first symptoms appear after a viral-like infection. The virus of infectious mononucleosis has been investigated, and discarded, as a cause. It was suspected in part because it was also a suspect in chronic fatigue syndrome (CFS), which is very similar to fibromyalgia. CFS, which in England is known as myalgic encephalomyelitis (ME), shares the fibromyalgia tender points, sleep disturbances and pain. Fatigue, however, predominates over pain, and patients often have low grade fever, sore throats and enlarged lymph glands – symptoms that suggest even more strongly an infectious cause.

The link is even more confusing in the case of Lyme disease – an infection caused by a spirochete passed on to humans by infected ticks (see next chapter). One of the symptoms of Lyme disease is arthritis. Unfortunately, Lyme disease is often very hard to diagnose. Symptoms may be confusing, and blood tests aren't reliable. Even in areas where Lyme disease is common, a positive result in a Lyme disease test is four times more likely to be false than true.

Recently, researchers in a Lyme disease clinic in Boston looked at musculoskeletal symptoms in all the patients they had been following for a number of years. The average follow-up was almost five years, which was sufficient time to be certain of the diagnosis. Almost half of their patients actually had Lyme disease, either active (23 percent) or inactive (20 percent). The rest (57 percent) had never had Lyme disease. What was startling was that in both groups, fibromyalgia or chronic fatigue syndrome was found in over half the patients. This suggests two things: (1) infection with Lyme disease may possibly trigger fibromyalgia, and (2) the symptoms of fibromyalgia may lead to a false diagnosis of Lyme disease. Certainly many people with fibromyalgia have been treated with repeated courses of antibiotics in a futile attempt at curing Lyme disease.

Human immunodeficiency virus (HIV) infection has also been linked to a high frequency of fibromyalgia symptoms.

Other types of arthritis, if they go on long enough, can lead to fibromyalgia on top of the original problem. This is fairly common in rheumatoid arthritis (RA), where shoulder pain often makes sleep very difficult. It makes sense that this might cause the kind of sleep disturbance that Smythe and Moldofsky provoked by slightly rousing volunteers in a sleep lab. When a patient with RA is feeling worse, it's important to recognize whether the problem is fibromyalgia. It's not a good idea to treat the wrong disease.

Abnormalities of pain perception may lie at the root of fibromyalgia, which has been called a "pain amplification syndrome." When pain sensation is tested in areas away from the 18 "tender points," people with fibromyalgia are much more sensitive than others. And when patients with fibromyalgia are asked to rate their pain on a 1 to 10 scale, and they are compared to patients with rheumatoid arthritis, their pain intensity is twice as high. Researchers have found several abnormalities that may explain the heightened sensitivity to pain experienced by people with fibromyalgia. Elevated levels of substance P (a chemical involved in pain transmission) have been found in cerebrospinal fluid – the fluid that bathes the brain and spinal cord. They have also documented relative deficiencies of serotonin – another chemical of the nervous system – and subnormal adrenal-gland hormone secretion in response to stress.

There are many – doctors, insurance company executives

and even one Canadian judge – who don't believe in fibromyalgia. Some see it as a psychiatric disorder, or as conscious malingering. I'm not in that camp. I've seen too many people – emotionally stable, hard-working, with nothing to gain and everything to lose – who have been laid low by fibromyalgia. I believe that, in time, the roots of the problem will be laid bare, and when that happens we will finally have an effective treatment approach.

How Is It Treated?
Whenever there's a long list of possible treatments for any disorder, you can be sure that none is very good. This is certainly true for fibromyalgia. There is no cure. The goal is to regain control, as much as possible, of a normal life.

Aerobic Fitness Conditioning
This is used because people with fibromyalgia are generally very unfit – probably as a result of their disease. Improving fitness does result in reduced pain, but it's not known if this effect will hold up over the long run. Most treatment programs combine fitness conditioning with muscle strengthening and general flexibility exercises. Twenty minutes of each – for a total of one hour – three times a week has been shown to improve the overall level of function. But this regimen must be built up to slowly and painstakingly. Ideally, an experienced physiotherapist should guide the patient along. Postural awareness and correction of bad postural habits can also be taught by the physiotherapist.

Tricyclics
Having recognized that sleep disturbance may be important in fibromyalgia, Smythe and Moldofsky tried a number of drugs that might affect sleep, and settled on amitriptyline.

Given in doses much lower than usually used in depression, amitriptyline is very effective in about a third of patients. The majority aren't helped, though. Those that do notice improvement often stop the drug because of unpleasant side effects such as feeling "zonked out" the next morning, or experiencing constipation or severe dryness of the mouth. Some of those who do carry on find that amitriptyline loses its initial benefit after a while. A number of related compounds, including cyclobenzaprine, give similar, rather disappointing results.

Avoidance of Inactivity

The other main benefit of an exercise program is to show patients with fibromyalgia that they can exercise and become fit, although their pain and fatigue tell them the opposite. By avoiding physical activity they become less and less fit, so they get caught up in a vicious circle of pain and fatigue leading to inactivity and deconditioning, which results in even more pain and fatigue. It's much like the situation of patients with chronic back pain; resting to relieve the pain is exactly the wrong thing to do.

Sleep Improvement

Better sleep can be expected with both tricyclic medication and fitness conditioning. Small things, such as changing to a smaller, molded pillow to support the head and neck in a neutral position, are often surprisingly helpful.

Stress Management

Stress is often a major part of the problem, and not just a result of fibromyalgia. It may in fact play a role in its development. Financial worries and abusive marital relationships are surprisingly common among patients. Counseling from an appropriate source, such as a social worker, may be a key element in coping with fibromyalgia.

Learning about Fibromyalgia

It's essential that Mary Jane understand her disease if she is going to keep it from controlling her life. The first step is the diagnosis. She needs to learn that the problem is not "all in her head," nor will it cripple or kill her. She needs to learn to recognize the various symptoms and not be frightened by them. She must realize that initial attempts at becoming more fit are going to be hard, and possibly even painful, but that in the long run they will pay off.

One of the best ways to learn about fibromyalgia is to link up with a group with the same problem. There are self-help groups devoted to fibromyalgia in many communities. The Arthritis Foundation (U.S.) and Arthritis Society (Canada) can provide more information.

Analgesics

Painkillers such as acetaminophen may be necessary and helpful, but NSAIDs don't work.

What's the Long-term Outlook?

This is a hard question to answer, because most patients have been looked at for only short periods. Also, studies have only been carried out in university centers, where the toughest cases are likely to be sent. Those, however, suggest that there is very little change, at least over the short term. At four-year and five-year follow-ups less than a quarter of the patients were better, and most were worse. Those who tended to improve were younger, and had had less overall pain to start with, than those who didn't.

Fibromyalgia seen outside these university centers may be much more benign – that's certainly the case with many other diseases. We know that the vast majority of patients continue to work full time, and those who aren't working should try to return to work. This may require the intensive combined efforts of doctor, physiotherapist and occupational therapist, as well as cooperation from the employer. But the result will be worth the hard and often painful effort.

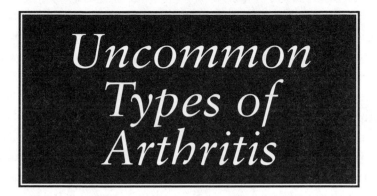

Uncommon Types of Arthritis

Lyme Disease

From time to time I see a patient who is very frightened. The patient invariably has the diffuse aches and pains characteristic of fibromyalgia. She or he has heard about Lyme disease, recalls a hiking or camping trip and may even have had a test for Lyme disease, which may or may not have been positive. Some have, in fact, been treated with antibiotics – unsuccessfully.

Why this extraordinary fear? It is probably due to several factors. First of all, Lyme disease is something new and it's infectious. Patients have heard that it can be serious, and that it can be hard to diagnose. Its symptoms can be confused with symptoms of other conditions. Lab tests may not always give clear-cut answers. And there is concern that a delay in treatment may have serious consequences.

Each of these points deserves comment. First, though, I'd like to tell the story of how Lyme disease came to be discovered.

In November of 1975, Polly Murray made an appointment to see Dr. Allen Steere, a Yale University medical scientist. She was an artist and mother of four living in Lyme, Connecticut, and for ten years she had been experiencing mysterious and unexplained symptoms – recurring fatigue, depression, weight loss and low-grade fevers. Several times she had attacks of joint pain and swelling. Doctors (she had been examined by many) were unable to explain her symptoms. It had even been suggested that the problem was "in her head." But in the months before her appointment with Dr. Steere, Mrs. Murray's husband and two of her children developed similar symptoms. She asked around, and discovered others in her community who seemed to be affected. By the time she met with Dr. Steere she had a list of 35 people who had been variously diagnosed with infectious arthritis, systemic lupus erythematosus, rheumatoid arthritis and juvenile rheumatoid arthritis. She was convinced that all had the same condition, and it was due to exposure to some common agent.

Dr. Steere believed Mrs. Murray, and within several months had identified, in Lyme and in two nearby communities, a total of 39 children and 12 adults who appeared to be suffering from some form of epidemic arthritis. The observation that most cases of arthritis came on in the summer months, and that for many the arthritis had been preceded by a rash resembling one known in Europe to be caused by a tick bite, pointed the search in the right direction. The story unfolded slowly, but by 1981 it was evident that Lyme disease:

- is an infection caused by a microscopic organism
- is passed on to humans by ticks
- can be successfully treated with antibiotics
- often starts with a typical skin rash, and can progress to involve the nerves, heart and/or joints

Even in southern Ontario, where I live – where possibly a dozen cases of Lyme disease have been convincingly proved – I am often asked, "Could I have Lyme disease?"

The Risk of Exposure to Lyme Disease

Lyme disease is caused by an organism that is transmitted to humans by the bite of the Ixodes tick. The species of Ixodes tick that carries this spirochete varies with the geographic location, but in New England it is *Ixodes dammini*. Initially this species was near extinction, found only on the island of Nantucket. The appearance of Lyme disease along the eastern seaboard corresponded to a tick population explosion, undoubtedly helped by its natural hosts, deer and the white-footed mouse. Since humans, mice and deer are increasingly neighbors, particularly as suburbia spreads in the heavily populated coastal corridor from Massachusetts to North Carolina, it's not surprising that occasionally an infected tick bites a human.

Lyme disease, and the Ixodes tick, appear to be spreading further and further each year. Some suspect that, in addition to being carried by deer and mice, the tick may be hitch-hiking on migrating birds.

The American seaboard states from Massachusetts to Maryland account for 75 percent of the more than 10,000 cases reported each year in the U.S. Most of the rest are in the northern Midwest (especially Minnesota and Wisconsin) and coastal West (particularly California). However, patients with Lyme disease have turned up in every state. Usually this is because they have vacationed in a "hot" or endemic area. Nevertheless, "native cases" do occur, even in Canada. Lyme disease is also found throughout most of Europe and northern Asia.

What Lyme Arthritis Looks Like

Soon after the bite, about the time the Lyme skin rash (described below) appears and for up to a month or two afterward, patients may experience muscular and joint aches and pains that move about the body without joint swelling.

The Good News about Lyme Disease

The Ixodes tick is very small, and may escape detection. But it isn't easy to catch Lyme disease; the tick must remain attached from 36 to 48 hours to pass on the infection. It has been estimated that even in those areas where up to 40 percent of all ticks are infected, only about 1 percent to 3 percent of tick bites will result in Lyme disease. With odds like that, a person bitten by a tick in an endemic area and treated with antibiotics "just in case" is far more likely to get sick from the treatment than from Lyme disease. And people themselves have to be bitten by the tick to be at risk. Although dogs can get Lyme disease, they never pass it on to their owners.

Lyme arthritis develops, on average, about six months after the initial tick bite. About 50 percent of those who acquire the infection develop arthritis. Lyme arthritis is quite obvious – the joint involved becomes very swollen and painful. Only one or two joints at a time are affected, and they tend to be large joints, particularly the knees. An affected joint will "cool off" after days to weeks, but it's common for another (or the same) joint to flare up again later. If the infection is not treated, attacks of single-joint arthritis tend to recur at increasing intervals, each attack just a bit less "hot" than the last, until, sometime within two to three years after the initial tick bite, no more attacks occur. Even if the patient is adequately treated and the infection cured, it may take several months for the arthritis attacks to wind down.

It's very rare for local inflammation to persist in a joint, and even more uncommon for bone and cartilage damage to develop. In a group of patients diagnosed with Lyme arthritis in the days before antibiotics were known to be effective, only 10 percent went on to chronic arthritis. In some of these patients, persisting infection may not be the problem. The infection may have triggered the initial arthritis, been eliminated by antibiotics but somehow initiated a process similar to reactive arthritis. In such cases, antimalarials and surgical removal of the inflamed joint tissue through an arthroscope have been used successfully.

Lyme arthritis never looks like rheumatoid arthritis, but it can look like one form of childhood arthritis.

As described in the preceding chapter, many people with Lyme disease develop symptoms that are classic for fibromyalgia. This poses a problem, because fibromyalgia itself is so common. How can we tell if fibromyalgia symptoms in a given patient are a consequence of Lyme disease? For one thing, we can consider the odds; even where Lyme disease is most commonly seen, fibromyalgia is still far more frequent. We can also take a careful history of exposure and symptoms, and consider the timing of the patient's symptoms when reviewing the results of blood testing. Fibromyalgia symptoms do not mean that the Lyme infection is active, and they do not respond to Lyme disease treatment with antibiotics.

Evidence of Lyme Disease Elsewhere in the Body

In about 5 percent of cases, arthritis is the first sign of Lyme disease, and sometimes it's the only one. The initial tick bite may not even be remembered – only about a third of patients recall being bitten. A correct diagnosis is therefore easier if other symptoms have been noticed.

The skin rash of Lyme disease, which follows the infected tick bite only 50 to 70 percent of the time, is called erythema chronicum migrans (ECM). It starts off as a small red bump where the tick has bitten – usually in the area of the armpit, groin or thigh. Over a few days it spreads outward in a rapidly enlarging circle, which may be several inches across. The center tends to clear as the red spot enlarges, giving the appearance of a "bull's eye." Without treatment, the rash clears within several days to weeks. Because it doesn't itch or hurt, if it's tucked away on the back or in the armpit it may not even be noticed.

The heart is affected in 5 to 10 percent of untreated patients. Symptoms may be absent, or there may be heart rhythm irregularities (palpitations). Dizziness and fainting spells may occur. These symptoms rarely last more than a few weeks.

Nervous system symptoms, which occur in about 10 percent of Lyme patients, may suggest infection of the brain (meningitis and encephalitis), spinal cord and major nerves in hands and feet. Headache, neck stiffness, difficulty concentrating and emotional upset can dominate the picture. There can be numbness, pain or weakness in the limbs. One very common symptom is the development of Bell's palsy: the nerve to half the face is affected, and that side of the face appears flattened. The corner of the mouth may droop and the smile is distinctly crooked. These symptoms tend to come on two to three months after the skin rash.

Heart and nervous system symptoms get better with treatment, although it may take several months for things to get completely back to normal.

Blood Tests for Lyme Disease

Blood tests will be negative for the first two to three weeks, and for up to eight weeks in some cases. Blood tests aren't necessary, however, if the evidence is there. If some or all of the clues fit – typical skin rash, memory of a tick bite, presence in an area of known Lyme disease and potential exposure to a tick, and symptoms consistent with Lyme disease – the diagnosis can be made.

Many people test positive for Lyme disease who have never had the disease. About 7 percent of the general public will have a positive ELISA test (to screen for Lyme exposure), whereas, even in areas where Lyme disease is most frequent, only 1 percent of tests are true positives. Other infections, mononucleosis, even rheumatoid arthritis, are among the many causes of a positive ELISA. On the other hand, a negative test means just that: the patient does not have, and never has had, Lyme disease, unless the test is done within eight weeks of the bite, or the patient has had antibiotics early in the disease. In the latter case the antibiotics may not have cured the disease, but the test may still be a false negative.

If a patient has a positive ELISA test and the picture is suspicious, a second test – the more specific Western blot test – is done. It too can be negative if done too soon or if the patient has been given antibiotics early on. A positive test isn't the end of it, though. It can give several different answers, all considered "positive" – but only if the particular answer exactly matches the patient's story.

What's a Patient to Do?

Where the probability of Lyme disease is high, it should be treated with antibiotics. High probability situations exist where there is a reasonable chance of past exposure to the Ixodes tick, where symptoms are consistent with Lyme disease, and where the blood test results fit the picture. Treatment isn't simple. It may involve intravenous antibiotics over three to four weeks.

Where the probability of Lyme disease is low – where a definite diagnosis of the disease has been appropriately treated but the patient continues to be tired, with aches and pains, or where a mistaken diagnosis of Lyme is made based on misinterpreted symptoms and lab tests – the risk of "pseudo-Lyme" is high. The patient and/or the doctor becomes convinced that Lyme disease is the problem. The result – according to one U.S. report – is repeated, unnecessary doctor visits, blood tests, courses of antibiotic treatment, side effects of treatment (in up to half the cases), time off work, depression and stress.

Prevention of Lyme Disease

The first step is common sense, especially in areas with infected ticks. Avoid woods and brushy areas in the late spring and early summer, when the ticks are most likely to attach. Wear light-colored long-sleeved garments, and tuck pants into socks. Inspect yourself or your child carefully, at night before the bath. Any attached ticks should be removed, after cleansing the skin with alcohol, with tweezers or gloved fingers. Don't dig out any mouth parts that remain embedded in the skin – they will be shed in a day or two. And don't forget – a tick has to be attached for more than a day to transmit the disease, and only 1 percent to 3 percent of tick bites in areas where Lyme is common actually result in the disease.

There is now a very effective vaccine against Lyme disease but, like all vaccines, it is not guaranteed to be 100 percent effective. And it only protects against Lyme. Many infected ticks carry other organisms, and the vaccine doesn't prevent the illnesses they cause. So, while it may make very good sense to vaccinate – especially children in areas where Lyme disease is common – it's also good sense to keep up measures to prevent and detect tick attachment.

Arthritis in Children

Arthritis in children is really quite uncommon, but it can occur for about as many different reasons as it occurs in adults. Whenever arthritis suddenly develops, whether in a child or an adult, a number of possibilities, such as infection and malignancy, have to be ruled out first. Once that's done, we are left with the problem of chronic arthritis.

In the United States, the term used is juvenile rheumatoid

arthritis (JRA). In Great Britain, the term is juvenile chronic arthritis (JCA). I prefer the British usage, because rheumatoid arthritis is only a small part of the overall picture of arthritis in children.

Varieties of Childhood Arthritis

Arthritis in children usually fits into one of three categories:

- arthritis involving relatively few joints
- arthritis involving many joints
- arthritis as part of Still's disease

Arthritis Involving Relatively Few Joints

Doctors call this "pauciarticular arthritis" ("pauci" means "few"), and it's the most common of the three. About 55 to 75 percent of childhood arthritis fits into this category.

Four or fewer joints are affected at any one time, and they tend to be larger joints – a knee, ankle or elbow. Occasionally small hand joints will also be affected.

Typically, the child is a girl and is under five years old when the problem begins. Pain may not be very obvious. In fact, up to a quarter of these children don't complain of pain. The first thing noticed may be that the child is limping, or is unable to straighten out the leg. The child is usually not otherwise ill. Blood tests for arthritis are negative except for the antinuclear antibody test (ANA), which is commonly positive and is an important marker for this disease.

Melanie was 17 when I first met her. She had a swollen knee which had been bothering her, off and on, for six years. This hadn't prevented her from trying to lead a normal life, and she was in fact a year ahead of her age group in school. What was remarkable was that she had done this despite being legally blind. Slowly and insidiously, beginning in her early teens, she had lost her vision.

Children with arthritis are at high risk of "silent" progressive eye damage, because of continuing low-grade inflammation in the front portion of the eye. The eye isn't red or painful, but the inflammation, called iridocyclitis, can cause cataracts, glaucoma, scarring of the cornea and loss of vision. The earliest signs can only be detected by careful examination by an eye specialist. Early detection, and the possibility of effective treatment, means that every child at risk must be followed carefully and frequently – at least annually into adulthood. The highest risk is within the first few years, and examinations should be more frequent then. Eye inflammation may occur, or progress, even if the joint disease is in remission.

When older children develop pauciarticular arthritis, it may be an indication that they will go on to develop ankylosing spondylitis, the arthritis of inflammatory bowel disease or psoriatic arthritis. Unlike the younger children, who almost never have hip arthritis, hip inflammation is common in this group.

Arthritis Involving Many Joints
About 20 percent of children with arthritis have polyarticular disease. By definition, five or more joints are affected. The arthritis may look a great deal like adult rheumatoid arthritis (RA), and roughly half of these children will have a positive test for rheumatoid factor (RF). As in adult RA, a positive RF test tends to identify those who are not going to do well over the long term; those with RF-negative polyarthritis do much better.

Arthritis As Part of Still's disease
A hundred years ago, George Frederic Still, a young English doctor in training, described the first cases of what has since

become known as Still's disease. Children with this variant make up about a fifth of all cases of childhood arthritis.

These children are sick, and look sick. They have a systemic (that is, involving many parts of the body) illness. High fevers, a blotchy red skin rash that comes and goes, enlarged lymph glands and a high white blood cell count often lead the doctor to search first for infection or childhood leukemia. Arthritis tends to appear later, developing in about three-quarters of patients within 3 to 12 months.

Attacks with the systemic features are unpredictable, varying from a single episode to recurring episodes over a number of years. Usually, however, this aspect of Still's disease subsides within five years. The arthritis, however, continues as a progressive illness in about half the cases. The more joints are involved, and the earlier the age of onset of Still's, the poorer the long-term outlook for full functioning as an adult.

Children with Still's disease sometimes die, with liver disease and infection the most common causes of death in North America. The heart may be involved, and heart failure can occur, particularly if there is severe anemia as well. The majority of deaths occur within the first 10 years of the illness.

What Happens in the Long Run?
A significant minority of children – 30 to 50 percent – experience abnormalities of growth. In many this seems to reflect the intense local inflammatory process. In the knee of a child of three or four, for example, the inflammation may provoke a "growth spurt" of the adjacent bones, and that leg may be longer as a result. In an older child, the same stimulus may cause a brief growth spurt and then early bone fusion at the growth center; since the opposite leg continues to grow, the affected leg will soon be shorter. Children who habitually don't use a leg because of pain may also show growth retardation in that leg.

About a fifth of children will have "micrognathia" (the jaw will be small and underdeveloped). Two patients I've been following since they were infants are now young women in their 20s; both have undergone jaw surgery to correct their "receding chin" deformity and improve the way their teeth come together, and both are delighted with the result.

Children who are sick with Still's disease will experience slowing of their growth as long as the disease is active, so an experienced child rheumatologist will monitor growth very carefully. Growth retardation is also seen in children who are put on corticosteroids such as prednisone. Since these drugs can also cause osteoporosis in both children and adults, they are used only after careful consideration of the risks, and measures are taken to reduce those risks.

Remission of the Arthritis

One of the cruel misconceptions about childhood arthritis is that the child will outgrow the disease. In fact, in just under half the children, the arthritis will continue past puberty.

The pattern of arthritis tends to stay the same over the years. Most of the children with pauciarticular arthritis will continue in that pattern; they have little disability and tend to do very well. For this group, vision is the big concern. However, some of them (about 15 percent) will evolve into a polyarticular pattern and won't do so well. The change from pauciarticular to polyarticular, if it is going to occur, usually happens within the first five years.

Half the children who have polyarticular disease and are RF-negative will do well, and even go into permanent remission. Similarly, half of those with Still's disease will experience remission. The other half, along with those with RF-positive polyarticular disease, are not so lucky, and most will develop major difficulties with functioning as the years go by. A very small number of children with polyarticular disease will have their eyes affected, so they too should be closely watched. It is very rare for the eye to be affected in Still's disease.

How Is Childhood Arthritis Treated?

Exactly the same principles of treatment that we use in adult arthritis apply here. They include:

- suppression of inflammation
- control of pain
- maintenance of function
- avoidance of complications

Because the long-term outlook in an individual child can only be guessed at, treatment is long-term and involves many

---

Dealing with Childhood Arthritis

Dr. Helen Emery, a San Francisco pediatric rheumatologist, sets out the following important principles:

- growth is a good indication of how well the disease is being controlled
- it's easy to treat a chronically ill child like an infant, but it's wrong
- keep the child in school. Schooling at home is often second-rate, and socialization suffers
- be aggressive with physiotherapy and occupational therapy. Be alert for joint contractures ("tightening up," especially of knee and hip), and treat them early
- be aware of the effect of the illness on the child, the parents, brothers and sisters. There are childhood arthritis telephone support groups, and summer camps for children with arthritis, and social workers and psychologists are available
- keep a balance. The child's life and the family's life should not revolve around the disease.

Finally, declares Dr. Emery,
- a child goes in a wheelchair over my dead body

different types of therapists. Pediatric rheumatologists, physiotherapists, occupational therapists, social workers and the family doctor make up the core team. Eye specialists, orthopedic surgeons, dietitians, psychologists and teachers are involved from time to time.

The drugs we use in children, particularly NSAIDs, gold, antimalarials, sulfasalazine and methotrexate, are virtually the same as those used in adults. Corticosteroid injections into joints may be particularly helpful. Children are not just little adults, of course, and special care has to be taken to ensure that the dose of each medication is appropriate and that monitoring for side effects is carried out.

Polymyositis and Dermatomyositis

"Myositis" means inflammation of muscle. "Dermato-" refers to an additional component of skin inflammation, and "poly-" means "many."

These two rare conditions – polymyositis is about twice as common as dermatomyositis – are similar in terms of who's affected to many of the other inflammatory diseases; women are more commonly affected, and the age of onset is usually between 40 and 60. A small number of children also develop the condition.

Sometimes these conditions develop in people who have other "connective tissue" diseases, particularly systemic lupus erythematosus. In a few patients, particularly those who are older when the symptoms develop, muscle inflammation may be a clue to an unsuspected cancer.

Signs and Symptoms of Polymyositis and Dermatomyositis

The main symptom is muscle weakness. It usually comes on very slowly, and is painless. At most, there is mild muscle aching. The muscles around the hips and the shoulders are those mainly affected. Patients have difficulty getting out of a chair, or off the toilet. Climbing stairs becomes difficult. Holding the arms up to shampoo hair or to hang clothes on a line becomes impossible. The neck muscles may become weak, and swallowing may be difficult.

If a skin rash develops, we call the condition dermatomyositis. The rash can be extensive; it's reddish in color, and in areas there may be thickening and scaling of the skin – particularly on the backs of the hands, mainly over the knuckles. Around the eyes the skin may have a purplish color.

Many patients will have systemic symptoms, such as fever, fatigue and weight loss. A number will have Raynaud's phenomenon – whitening of the fingers with exposure to cold. Shortness of breath may develop, due to one or more factors: the breathing muscles may be weak, there may be inflammatory scarring in the lungs and in some individuals the heart muscle itself is affected.

There has been a great deal of debate over whether the disease is linked to cancer. There is general consensus that it is, since cancer is more common in patients with dermato/polymyositis than in patients of similar background with rheumatoid arthritis, but not all researchers are convinced. In at least some instances polymyositis leads to discovery of a cancer, surgical removal results in marked improvement in the polymyositis and then the cancer and the polymyositis return together at a later date. As mentioned, the risk of cancer seems to be in the older age groups, especially in people with dermatomyositis. The cancer is usually obvious after a reasonable (not an exhaustive) investigation, and if it hasn't turned up within two to three years it probably won't.

Diagnosis

Diagnosis usually requires three separate approaches. Blood tests are done to detect elevated levels of enzymes released from the inflamed muscles. Electromyography (insertion of a fine needle into the muscle to measure electrical activity) gives additional information. Finally, the most important test is a muscle biopsy. A small sample of muscle is removed, either by surgery or through a large needle, and examined under the microscope. The first two tests are needed because the inflammatory process may be "patchy" (not evenly distributed in all muscles) and may come and go in intensity, so the muscle enzyme levels may sometimes be normal. The biopsy is done because there are other muscle diseases that may act the same, but look different under the microscope and respond quite differently to treatment.

Treatment

Initially, patients are treated with corticosteroids, usually prednisone, in high doses. They often feel better soon after treatment is started, but it may take up to three months for full muscle strength to return. Patients should also be put on preventive treatment for osteoporosis. High-dose steroids must be continued for some time – at least until the muscle enzyme level drops to normal. Thereafter, the dose is slowly reduced. Not all patients respond to this treatment, however, and sometimes it's necessary to add either methotrexate or azathioprine. Recently, intravenous treatment with gamma globulin has been shown to help in patients who still don't respond – but the only patient I used it on showed little obvious benefit.

Outcome

Treatment has improved the outlook substantially over the last 40 years. People still die, though, from infection or as a result of lung or heart involvement. My personal experience has varied. I am currently following two patients who have had the disease for well over 20 years. Both have stable but persisting weakness, and although they require continuing treatment they are able to live normal lives. I have had a number of patients whose treatment was stopped as they improved, and they remain well. But I have also had several patients whose polymyositis was linked to cancers that proved fatal.

Scleroderma (Systemic Sclerosis)

"Sclero-" means "hard," "-derma" refers to the skin. Scleroderma is a condition where the skin is tight and thickened. Its other name – "systemic sclerosis" – recognizes the fact that this process doesn't just involve the skin. Other parts of the body can also be affected.

This is a rare disease. Like many of the other so-called "autoimmune" or "connective tissue" disorders, it affects more women than men, and tends to come on in the 30s and 40s.

Skin Characteristics in Scleroderma

Early on, the skin involved (generally the skin of the hands and feet, and often the skin of the face) may be reddened and puffy. This period is brief, however, and in typical scleroderma the skin soon becomes tight and shiny. The fingers and hands are particularly affected. Wrinkles, and even the fine hairs on the backs of fingers, disappear. The skin on the back of the fingers resists pinching. Tightness restricts finger movement, and it's difficult to straighten fingers fully or make a fist. Fingertips are easily injured, and cracks may be slow to heal.

The extent of this change varies from patient to patient. In some it may be limited to the fingers and hand, in others it may involve the arm, face, trunk or legs. The process seems to spread from the fingers and toes, and move centrally.

Telangiectasia
Small blood vessels, normally invisible to the naked eye, often dilate enough to be apparent. Reddish "freckles" that briefly turn pale when pressed are common, particularly on the face and palms.

Raynaud's phenomenon
Fingers (and sometimes toes) turn dead white and numb with exposure to cold, and then experience burning, flushing and tingling when rewarmed. While Raynaud's is common in other conditions (and in up to 10 percent of the general population), here it is almost always present, probably reflecting the fact that circulation to the fingers is seriously reduced as part of the "tightening" process.

Systemic Involvement

Microscopic Thickening and Scarring of Lung Tissue
X-rays and pulmonary function tests show that well over half the patients with scleroderma do not have normal lungs. Many of them have no symptoms, but others experience shortness of breath, particularly with exercise.

The other lung complication that may develop is called "pulmonary hypertension." This isn't common, but it is serious: the prolonged effort of pumping blood into the arteries of the lungs may overload the capacity of the heart, and heart failure can result.

Heartburn
This is one of the most common systemic symptoms of scleroderma. The muscle of the esophagus (the passage from

throat to stomach) becomes thin and weak, and is largely replaced by scar tissue. This means that swallowing is inefficient and occasionally difficult, and that the acid contents of the stomach frequently flow back up the esophagus and cause pain. Scleroderma can also affect other parts of the gut. Constipation or diarrhea may become a problem.

Heart Involvement
This is not often a symptom but there can be thickening of the membrane around the heart (the pericardium), and occasionally it's inflamed and causes pain (pericarditis). Actual heart muscle is rarely involved, although there may be patchy scarring. High blood pressure and pulmonary hypertension can tax the heart's ability to pump effectively.

Scleroderma of the Kidney
This is also not very common, but it is extremely serious. It often develops quite suddenly, with severe high blood pressure and kidney failure. The initial problem seems to occur in the small blood vessels of the kidney. They narrow, choking off normal blood flow. This triggers a chemical release from the kidneys that causes severe hypertension. High blood pressure in turn causes further kidney blood vessel damage, and the vicious circle continues.

What Happens in the Long Term?
I diagnosed scleroderma in Jack four years ago and have been following him ever since. Tightening and stiffening of his fingers and hands, along with Raynaud's phenomenon, were what first brought him to me. He was 56, the manager of a local farm co-op, and I was pleased that my initial examination turned up nothing that would suggest a serious complication. I was wary, however, realizing that things could turn sour on fairly short notice. And that's exactly what happened.

Three days after I had checked him over, about a year into his illness, he was admitted to his local hospital with severe high blood pressure and kidney and heart failure. He was lucky: the problem was immediately recognized and he was transferred to the kidney unit and treated aggressively. He weathered the storm, but not without a price. He is now on dialysis three times weekly. His quality of life is surprisingly good. He's working full time, and I suspect that in the not too distant future he'll be lined up for a kidney transplant.

Generalizations are often untrustworthy, but one that seems to hold up pretty well is that the first two to three years are critical. If someone gets through this period without a major complication, the chances are one won't develop. In fact, in the long haul, some patients show definite improvement in the skin tightening. So the strategy is to watch the patient carefully, and to intervene quickly if complications such as high blood pressure develop.

At this time there is no treatment for either lung scarring or pulmonary hypertension. When patients develop symptoms of either, the outlook is poor.

Until a few years ago we thought the same about kidney involvement. The development of high blood pressure was an ominous sign. Treatment was generally ineffective, and these patients died of kidney failure. Today, however, a new class of antihypertensives, the ACE-inhibitors, is effective in arresting and even reversing high blood pressure and kidney failure in many people. Dialysis and transplant offer realistic alternatives if things reach the stage of kidney failure.

CREST

There is a form of localized scleroderma, known as CREST, which seems to have a better outlook. CREST is an acronym, and the letters stand for

Calcinosis – small calcium deposits, the size of clumps of salt crystals, scattered beneath the skin and detectable by X-ray

Raynaud's phenomenon

Esophagus involvement

Sclerodactyly – hardening of the skin of the fingers (and often very little more. No skin hardening above the elbow is allowed under this definition)

Telangiectasia – the little red "freckles" of dilated blood vessels

Individuals with CREST have a much lower risk of kidney involvement. Pulmonary hypertension, however, remains a definite concern.

Treatment of Scleroderma

Studies at the University of Pittsburgh have strongly suggested that D-penicillamine, a drug that interferes with the maturation of collagen (the protein chains that bind the skin down), influences the disease favorably.

None of the other drugs used has ever been shown to affect the disease course, although there is some enthusiasm for using methotrexate to intervene early on, in the "inflammatory" stage of scleroderma, when there is swelling and redness of the skin of the hands and face. Many doctors feel that this is the crucial stage, and that by the time the tight, hard skin develops the damage has already been done.

We need better means to identify early scleroderma, and more effective ways to arrest it. For now, we are left to deal with problems as they arise. This means

- watching carefully for the development of high blood pressure (which we can do something about)

- using physiotherapy to attempt to prevent contractures (stiffening up of the joints, which prevents full movement)
- dealing with heartburn with advice to avoid evening snacks and to elevate the head of the bed on blocks; drugs such as omeprazole may be necessary
- minimizing problems of reduced circulation to the hands and fingers by insisting on no smoking, encouraging warm mitts in the cold, and paying prompt attention to small nicks and cuts. Occasionally, drugs such as calcium-channel blocking agents marginally improve the finger circulation and help relieve the most intense symptoms of Raynaud's phenomenon.

Sjögren's Syndrome (Sicca Syndrome)

Dryness of the eyes and mouth may reflect aging and use of certain medications (particularly antidepressants). It is also a common feature of many of the autoimmune diseases, including rheumatoid arthritis, lupus erythematosus and scleroderma, where the dryness reflects inflammatory scarring of the glands that make lubricating tears and saliva.

This dryness often makes for intolerable eye itching or "grittiness." I often get my first clue that Sjögren's is a problem when patients volunteer that they use lubricating eye drops every day. I then ask if they keep a glass of water on the bedside table, if they wake up with their tongue stuck to the roof of the mouth, if they can chew and swallow a soda cracker without washing it down with a drink.

There are also situations where the inflammatory scarring of these glands appears to be unconnected to any other disease. In those cases, we speak of "primary" Sjögren's syndrome.

Primary Sjögren's (pronounced "show-grins") syndrome may have a variety of symptoms other than dryness. These include:

- episodic or persistent swelling of the parotid glands (the main source of saliva). These are located just in front of the ears, and swelling gives the cheeks a "chipmunk" look
- muscle and joint pains, and even joint swelling that may resemble rheumatoid arthritis, but does not result in cartilage or bone damage
- Raynaud's phenomenon

It has been discovered that a small number of people with primary Sjögren's syndrome (not those whose dryness is linked to other forms of arthritis) develop a form of lymph gland cancer. This is quite uncommon, but does mean that periodic follow-up visits are a good idea.

As in secondary Sjögren's syndrome – related to other arthritic conditions – the treatment of primary Sjögren's is symptomatic. Artificial tears, mouth lubricants, sugar-free gum and lemon drops help relieve dryness. Pilocarpine – a drug that stimulates the remaining glandular tissue to produce tears and saliva – is sometimes surprisingly effective. Careful attention to dental hygiene is important. Joint pain and swelling, and Raynaud's phenomenon, are also dealt with in their own right, symptomatically.

S I X

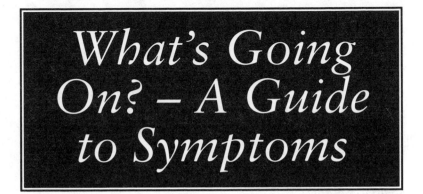

What's Going On? – A Guide to Symptoms

Patients with arthritis are often concerned about a new problem. Sometimes they can see a connection to their arthritis, but often they can't.

The following are some of the more common, or more important, symptoms that are linked to arthritis, organized by the areas where they tend to crop up. Some occur in many different kinds of arthritis, some are very disease-specific. Some are also found in people who are otherwise quite healthy.

Head and Neck
- headache
- scalp tenderness
- skin rash
- dry eyes (and often mouth)
- red, sometimes painful eyes
- changes in vision
- ear pain
- pain with chewing
- hoarseness and/or pain with swallowing
- neck pain

Headache

Headache is common as a symptom of neck arthritis, especially rheumatoid arthritis (RA) and osteoarthritis (OA). It's usually felt at the back of the skull, and may spread forward up and over the scalp to the sides and front. A good physiotherapist can help with advice, especially regarding neck support at night, the way to use ice and gentle movement exercises. Sometimes gentle traction and even local corticosteroid injection may be necessary.

Scalp Tenderness

When headache is coupled with scalp tenderness, the tenderness may be a clue to localized inflammation of one of the scalp blood vessels. This is called temporal (giant cell) arteritis; it's related to polymyalgia rheumatica and is potentially very serious. The headache is usually very localized, and is usually in the area of the temple. Tenderness when combing or brushing the hair may be the symptom that is most troublesome. In the most severe cases, inflammation of another artery, the one providing blood to the visual nerve, may cause sudden loss of vision.

Skin Rash

This is common in two kinds of arthritis. A red and sometimes scaling rash over the bridge of the nose, frequently much worse after being out in the sun, is characteristic of systemic lupus erythematosus (SLE). An itching, scaling, reddish rash in the hair at the back of the scalp – often ignored for years as "dandruff" – or behind the ears, or in the ear canal, may be the only proof that a patient with a single swollen joint has psoriatic arthritis.

Dry Eyes

Eye dryness leading to an itchy, "gritty" feeling is characteristic of Sjögren's syndrome. This happens in roughly 25 percent of people with RA, but is also seen in other arthritic conditions including SLE. It occurs just as often in people who have no arthritis. Dryness occurs because the tear gland of the eye is affected by low-grade inflammation, and tear production drops. Particular care has to be taken of the cornea, the clear membrane covering the pupil. It's much more easily scratched, especially by contact lenses, and if that happens it can become infected. Artificial tears, which can be bought at any drugstore, help restore lubrication to the eye, but they are never as good as the real thing.

People with Sjögren's syndrome (or "sicca syndrome") often also notice marked dryness of the mouth and, in the case of women, the vagina. Many patients use sugarless lemon drops or gum to stimulate saliva. I've never been very impressed with artificial mouth lubricants, but in the last few years a drug that stimulates the remaining glands to produce their own lubricant – pilocarpine – has become available in tablet form. I've been quite pleased with its effectiveness. Finally, without the protection of normal saliva the teeth are very vulnerable to cavities. It's important to brush and floss daily, and to get regular dental checks. The teeth can be protected by special applications of a fluoride solution.

Red, Sometimes Painful Eyes

These may be a sign of significant corneal damage in Sjögren's syndrome. They may also occur in RA (where the eye is usually painless) or in the seronegative forms of spondylarthritis (such as ankylosing spondylitis and psoriatic arthritis), where they may be quite irritable. Photophobia (discomfort from bright lights) can be a real problem. Red eyes tend to clear up, though an eye specialist should probably be consulted, especially if pain or blurring of vision occurs.

Changes in Vision

These are uncommon. Those that complicate the red eyes just mentioned tend to occur slowly. Even slower to develop is the "silent" loss of vision seen in some forms of childhood (juvenile chronic) arthritis – which is why monitoring by an eye specialist is so important. A sudden loss of vision, or double vision or blurring of vision, is a serious symptom of temporal arteritis. Antimalarial drugs should never lead to vision changes if taken as prescribed, although the eyes should still be checked by an eye specialist at least twice a year. Much more likely is the possibility of "speeded-up" development of cataracts when patients are on long-term corticosteroid treatment.

Ear Pain

This usually isn't from the ear itself. It may arise from arthritis in the jaw joint (temporomandibular joint, or TMJ), but is much more commonly from inside the mouth (such as an abscessed tooth) or the throat.

Pain with Chewing

If pain is felt just in front of the ear, it's almost certainly coming from the TMJ. If, however, a patient tells me the pain is in the temple region at the side of the skull, I think of temporal arteritis.

Hoarseness and/or Pain with Swallowing

Inflammatory arthritis – usually RA – can affect any joint in the body. That includes the tiny joints that anchor the vocal cords in the throat. Inflammation here can cause hoarseness, or pain in the throat with swallowing. This isn't common, but it may cause a lot of worry. Inhalable corticosteroid sprays, normally used in the treatment of asthma, are the most effective way to settle down the inflammation.

Neck Pain

Neck pain is very common – almost as common as low back pain. It comes on suddenly, causes severe pain with movement, responds to local ice and neck support (with a firm collar or soft "ruff") and clears up within days to a few weeks. Unlike low back pain, I would not recommend chiropractic manipulation for neck pain.

Most neck pain, though, spills over into the surrounding tissues, either up the back of the skull or down into the shoulder region. Neck pain may be referred from somewhere else, such as the heart. Heart attack pain, and similar referred pain, tends to be felt in the front or sides of the neck, whereas true neck pain tends to be felt in the muscles in the back of the neck.

A word about X-rays: just about everyone over the age of 40 will have a "terrible-looking neck" on X-ray. Don't take such a diagnosis seriously. If there is significant neck disease, a careful examination, which is a far better test, will pick it up.

Chest

- chest pain
- heart pain
- breastbone pain
- cough and/or shortness of breath

Chest Pain

Sharp, severe chest pain with breathing can be due to a "muscle pull" or a fractured rib, but most commonly it's a sign of inflammation of the pleural membrane. This membrane (actually two) consists of a thin double layer of tissue that surrounds the lungs. A very small amount of fluid coats the inner layer, and allows it to move gently and smoothly within the outer layer as the lungs expand and shrink with each breath.

Inflammation between these layers is called "pleurisy." Usually pleurisy is a symptom of lung infection, but it can also occur in arthritis – particularly in RA and SLE. If it does happen, and causes pain, treatment, usually with a brief course of corticosteroids, will settle things down.

Heart Pain

"Crushing" chest pain, felt front and center and sometimes also in the neck, jaw and/or left arm, is well known as the typical pain of a heart attack. What isn't so well known is that pericarditis (inflammation of the double-layered membrane that encloses the heart) can provoke pain that is identical.

The typical story goes something like this: "Right now I'm not having pain unless I cough or take a very deep breath, but last night I was really frightened. I woke up and it felt like someone was standing right in the middle of my chest. My jaw ached, and my left arm felt heavy and had a dull ache too. I felt really short of breath and sat up. That seemed to help the pain, but each time I lay back it got worse again."

Like pleurisy, pericarditis can be part of the inflammation of arthritis, and again, it usually happens in a patient with either RA or SLE. Again, corticosteroids, and sometimes NSAIDs, are helpful in relieving inflammation and pain.

Pericarditis does not mean that the heart has been damaged.

Breastbone Pain

Inflammatory arthritis, especially RA, may cause pain in the joints that connect the inner ends of the collar-bones (the clavicles) to the breastbone (the sternum). Pain and swelling will be noted on either side of the windpipe (the trachea) just as it disappears below the sternum. There is also a joint (the manubrio-sternal joint) in the breastbone, about three finger-breadths below the notch where the windpipe disappears, which can become inflamed. Finally, on either side of the sternum, where the ribs attach, tenderness (but not inflammation) is also common, particularly in fibromyalgia.

Cough and/or Shortness of Breath

Many forms of inflammatory arthritis – particularly RA – and many of the less common connective tissue disorders (such as dermatomyositis and scleroderma) can affect the lung. Microscopic scarring can occur, leading to shortness of breath with exertion and, often, a dry cough. Sometimes the problem is due to a build-up of fluid in the space between the two layers of tissue that surround the lung.

Shortness of breath is not a common symptom in arthritis, and it is always necessary to investigate it fully to be sure it isn't due to some other cause, such as infection. Some of the drugs used to treat arthritis may also turn out to be the culprit, so this symptom, although quite unusual in arthritis, should be reported.

Abdomen

- difficulty swallowing
- heartburn
- cramps, diarrhea
- black or bloody bowel movements

Difficulty Swallowing

Swallowing problems aren't common – if you don't count trying to get down all the pills some of you have to take each day. For that, it's useful to remember to swallow standing up, and to wash the pills down with a second glass of water.

If the muscles that control swallowing are carefully studied, using special techniques, muscle weakness or incoordination can be discovered in quite a number of people with some of the connective tissue disorders, particularly scleroderma (lupus and inflammatory muscle diseases are also in this category). This can lead to a feeling that food is "catching" behind the breastbone.

Heartburn

Heartburn (or reflux esophagitis) is the symptom of burning felt behind the breastbone, sometimes associated with a sour acid taste. It is particularly a problem at night, especially if the victim has eaten later in the evening. Sometimes the patient awakens choking. The acid stomach contents have not only come back up the esophagus (the "swallowing tube") from the stomach, but have spilled into the upper part of the breathing passages. Spasm of the larynx is brief, but can be very frightening.

This is a problem for many non-arthritics, particularly those who are overweight or pregnant. But the same muscle incoordination of the esophagus that slows swallowing in some forms of arthritis may also affect the valve at the opening of the esophagus into the stomach. This too allows "acid reflux" to occur.

The most effective treatment is to avoid food in the evening. Elevating the head of the bed on six-inch (15 cm) blocks, or placing a foam wedge under the mattress to raise the upper body, will work, but both are awkward. Sometimes a prescription medication to reduce stomach acid and improve the action of the valve is called for. Ranitidine seems to work well for most people.

Cramps, Diarrhea

These aren't usually symptoms of arthritis, unless there is an underlying problem of ulcerative colitis or Crohn's disease. Much more likely is the possibility that the problems are caused by medication. These symptoms should be reported to the doctor. If this isn't immediately possible, the next dose of the arthritis medicine (except corticosteroids) should be skipped until there has been an opportunity to sort out the problem.

Black or Bloody Bowel Movements
A bit of blood on the toilet paper is common and is usually a sign of unimportant bleeding, such as from a "pile," or hemorrhoid. But black bowel movements – assuming you haven't been taking iron pills or stomach medicines (like Pepto-Bismol) that contain bismuth, which create this effect – mean significant bleeding from higher up in the gastrointestinal tract. The most common source is an ulcer in either the stomach or the small intestine. The usual cause for this, in patients with arthritis, is medication – usually an NSAID.

Recognizable blood, either bright or dark red, usually means the bleeding is from lower down, often in the large intestine. However, if a stomach ulcer is bleeding briskly, the blood may travel down the intestinal tract so quickly that it doesn't have time to be chemically changed to the black color.

Whatever the cause, black or bloody bowel movements mean trouble. Get medical attention quickly.

Genitals
- discharge from the penis
- blood in the urine
- vaginal symptoms

Discharge from the Penis
There are two situations where this can be linked to arthritis. Gonorrhea, one of the sexually transmitted diseases, can cause an acute arthritis. The appearance of a hot and swollen

joint (often a wrist or knee) may in fact be the first indication that the symptoms of burning on urination and the slight discharge from the penis were important.

Reactive arthritis is discussed more fully elsewhere in this book. It too can be triggered by a sexually transmitted disease, such as chlamydia, and a discharge from the penis can precede its development.

Blood in the Urine

When blood is detected in the urine, it's usually microscopic blood, found in the course of a routine urine test; the urine sample is clear to the naked eye. When the urine is visibly pink or red, the bleeding is usually from the bladder, prostate, urethra or vagina, and is not related to either arthritis or its treatment. The one exception is an unusual one – when gout is complicated by the formation of kidney stones. Then the bleeding is invariably accompanied by "terrible" knifelike pain in the flank. This pain often spreads around from the back to the lower abdomen and into the groin. In men, it's often felt into the testicle.

Vaginal Symptoms

These too are not often related to arthritis. Vaginal dryness, which is common as part of Sjögren's syndrome, and vaginal ulcerations, which occasionally appear in lupus, are two exceptions. Gonorrhea, in women as in men, may cause an acute inflammatory arthritis, but it doesn't usually cause distinctive vaginal symptoms.

Lymph Nodes

Swollen "glands" in the neck, armpits and groin are often discovered accidentally. They don't usually cause discomfort. There are, of course, many reasons why lymph nodes become enlarged, and their discovery should be pointed out to your doctor. They are surprisingly common in rheumatoid arthritis, and are almost always benign. Nevertheless, enlarged lymph nodes may be an important sign of a completely different problem and should not be ignored.

Shoulder, Arm and Hand

- shoulder and arm pain
- elbow pain, lumps and swellings
- wrist pain at the base of the thumb
- numbness in the hands
- fingers that "lock"
- the suddenly droopy finger
- white fingers
- "funny" fingernails

Shoulder and Arm Pain
There are several possible causes of shoulder pain, but it usually isn't too hard to figure out the cause of most. It is important to get a precise description of the location of the pain itself, and then some idea of what makes it better or worse.

One principle that's important to remember: if the pain isn't affected by movement of the shoulder, it's probably coming from somewhere else.

Pain Originating in the Bones, Muscles or Nerves of the Neck
This is felt in the muscles on top of the shoulder, between the base of the neck and the end of the collarbone. It can also radiate upward into the back of the skull. If shoulder pain of this type is felt on one side only, it is almost certainly mechanical and not inflammatory in origin. If it involves both sides, either category is possible. If there's pressure on one of the nerves as it exits between the bones of the neck, shoulder pain

will track down the arm, and it can be accompanied by tingling or weakness in the arm and hand. Pain of this type will be aggravated by movement of the head and neck, and sometimes made better by such unusual "tricks" as placing the hand on top of the head.

Pain Originating at the Outside End of the Collarbone

Pain in the acromioclavicular joint, that is, where the outer end of the collarbone links up with the shoulder blade, is quite localized to that joint. You can feel the joint by tracing the collarbone out toward the point of the shoulder; it's just before the "bump" of the acromion (the bone that forms the tip of the shoulder), and you can identify it by rotating your arm at the shoulder joint. If this joint is the problem the pressure of your finger will cause pain, and you may feel a "grinding" as the shoulder moves around.

Pain from the Shoulder Joint Itself, or from the Tendons and Ligaments That Surround It (the "Rotator Cuff")

This is often felt not in the shoulder but in the upper outer arm, about three inches below the tip of the shoulder. Pain here is much worse if the arm is raised sideways to the horizontal, and may be so sharp that lowering the arm slowly back down is impossible. Halfway down, if there is a tear or a painful focus in the rotator cuff, you will be forced to let the arm fall limply to your side. Shoulder pain of this type can usually be traced to inflammation of a bursa (see below) or tendon just beneath the acromion. It is common in many forms of arthritis, but is even more common in "normal" people. There isn't much room between the acromion and the head of the humerus (the part of the arm bone that links up to form the shoulder joint), and shoulder movement narrows the gap even more. Shoulder tendons, and the bursa that cushions them, fill this gap and are easily inflamed by overuse. Pain is particularly bad at night. NSAIDs, and in resistant cases local corticosteroid injections, usually settle the problem.

Pain "Referred" to the Arm or Shoulder from Somewhere Else
Referred pain is characteristically from a source deep in the body. The brain has difficulty "reading" its source, and is tricked by the nervous system into mislabeling it. The best-known example is the pain when the oxygen supply to the heart is insufficient. The pain of angina is often felt as a deep ache in the entire left arm, worse with excitement or exertion and better with rest. Pain from the part of the abdomen beneath the diaphragm may be felt on top of the shoulder, just above the shoulderblade. This may, in fact, be the first sign of a gall bladder attack.

Elbow Pain, Lumps and Swellings
Elbow pain may be due to joint disease, but the most common cause is epicondylitis. When it's on the outside of the elbow the popular term is "tennis elbow," and when it's on the inside the term is "golfer's elbow." Pain is felt at, or just below, one of the bony bumps at the elbow. The two outer bumps are the epicondyles. The one in the middle (at the point of the elbow) is the olecranon; if it's tender, bursitis (see below) may be the problem.

There's some argument as to what is actually going on, but there's no disagreement as to the location. Pain arises in the area where the forearm muscle tendons attach to the elbow. In the case of "tennis elbow" the muscles are those that brace the wrist when you make a tight fist (as in holding a tennis racket). The opposing muscles, those that hold the wrist in the slightly bent position, cause pain on the inside of the elbow when contracted. Age (over 40) and overuse (most cases are not caused by tennis or golf) are felt to be the main factors in development of epicondylitis. There have been over 40 different treatments proposed, but the injection of corticosteroid clears up the symptoms in almost everyone. To be honest, however, most patients (if willing to be patient) will recover on their own within the next 12 months.

Common swellings of the elbow region

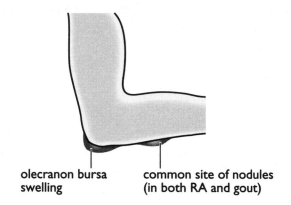

olecranon bursa   common site of nodules
swelling   (in both RA and gout)

In addition to swelling of the elbow joint itself (which makes it impossible to fully bend or straighten the arm), there are at least two fairly common types of swelling in this region:

- bursitis
- rheumatoid nodules

A bursa is a small, collapsed sac containing a few drops of lubricating fluid – think of an uninflated balloon. The body has many bursae which lie particularly at pressure points, where they cushion the skin from being damaged by local injury. The olecranon bursa sits under the skin just below the tip of the elbow, at the point where we usually rest our elbows on the arms of a chair. Fluid accumulation can swell the balloon, and then the bursa can be felt as quite puffy and sometimes tense.

Sudden swelling is painful. It can be caused by injury (a fall on an icy sidewalk), inflammation (gout can do it) or infection. If there is any doubt, check it out with a doctor.

Slower swelling is usually painless. The bursa is less puffy, but it's constantly getting in the way. This type of swelling has a number of possible causes. Local injury is probably the most common. It's very often seen, however, in rheumatoid arthritis.

It's usual to make sure that infection isn't the problem. If there's any doubt a sample of fluid is drained off through a needle and sent to the lab. Once infection has been ruled out, the bursa is left alone. If local injury caused it, it will go down on its own. Cortisone injections tend to speed up the process and have been used where rheumatoid arthritis is the cause, with some success and some failures. If the bursa doesn't settle down then, and its size is a problem, it is sometimes removed surgically.

Rheumatoid nodules are similar in that they can be removed but will often return. They are most often found just below the elbow, on the forearm where it rests on the arms of a chair. Such nodules can develop in a number of other locations – all it takes is rheumatoid arthritis (and usually rheumatoid factor) and pressure. Nodules on fingers, over knuckles or where a pencil or a hammer is held tightly, and on the back of the heel where the shoe or boot rubs, are almost as common. They are usually small – pea-sized or less.

Wrist Pain at the Base of the Thumb

There are two sources of pain here.

One is osteoarthritis between one of the wrist bones and the thumb metacarpal. This is common, particularly in the non-dominant hand (in most of us, the left hand). It shows up as aching, and sharp pain with tight gripping, and in time a bony lump often develops over this joint. Local cortisone injection, a thumb splint or, very rarely, surgery are ways to deal with this.

The other is de Quervain's tenosynovitis – inflammation of the tendon that pulls the thumb back in a "hitch-hiking" position. NSAIDs and splinting may help, but if the inflammation persists a local cortisone injection may be needed.

Numbness in the Hands

About 1 in every 1,000 adults has this problem at any given time. The usual story is something like this: "What's wrong with my hand? I'm waking up every night with burning pain in my fingers. They feel numb, especially my thumb and the next three fingers. If I hang my arm over the side of the bed, or shake my hand hard, the numbness improves and I can get back to sleep. It comes on during the day too, especially if I'm holding up a newspaper or gripping the steering wheel for a long time."

The diagnosis here is "carpal tunnel syndrome," and the problem is pressure on the median nerve at the wrist. The median nerve is responsible for sensation in the palm side of the thumb and the first three fingers. This nerve also causes the muscle in the palm, at the base of the thumb, to contract.

Pressure can be due to many things, including some that have nothing to do with arthritis (pregnancy and low thyroid function are just two). But in my practice RA is the most common cause. Median nerve pressure is caused by inflammatory swelling of the tissues at the wrist that lie just beneath the nerve. The nerve gets trapped between this swollen tissue and the tough ligament that crosses above it. When the nerve is injured in this fashion, patients hurt.

Wrist anatomy in carpal tunnel syndrome

An occupational therapist can provide the patient with a carpal tunnel splint to wear at night. This keeps the wrist from bending and putting even more pressure on the nerve.

If symptoms are really severe and medical management appears ineffective, surgery is recommended. (If symptoms persist for too long, the nerve can be permanently damaged.) Pressure can be relieved permanently by a relatively simple surgical procedure, "carpal tunnel release," which involves cutting the restraining ligament. This is often done on an outpatient basis, with the patient going home the same day.

Fingers That "Lock"

Rheumatologists call this a "trigger finger." It's fairly common, and it's due to inflammatory thickening on one of the tendons that bend the fingers. This thickening, like a knot in a rope, blocks the smooth flow of the tendon as the finger muscles contract. The knot gets stuck, or catches on corners. This is easy to treat. An injection of a corticosteroid in the thickened area usually frees things up.

The Suddenly Droopy Finger

The extensor tendons of the fingers (those on the back of the hand, which allow us to point fingers at others) pass through some tissue at the back of the wrist called the "tenosynovial sheath." This tissue is often inflamed, swollen and painful in RA, and the inflammation can thin and weaken the tendons. A sudden "ping," a sharp pain, and a finger droops. Considering how common this type of swelling is, it's surprising that tendon rupture doesn't happen more often. Sometimes a surgeon removes the inflamed tissue if wrist pain on finger movement suggests that tendon rupture is likely. Usually, however, surgery occurs after the event. The tendon is reattached or replaced and the inflammatory tissue removed.

White Fingers

The story here is usually "Every time I go out in the cold without my gloves, my fingers go white. I lose the feeling in them. When I warm them up they go purple, then fiery red, and they burn for several minutes." Sometimes the simple act of scrubbing potatoes under the cold-water tap, or jumping into Lake Huron in July, will have the same effect.

This is Raynaud's phenomenon. It's very common, particularly in young women. Approximately 10 percent of the population report Raynaud's symptoms, and most of the time they don't signify an underlying problem. Raynaud's can, however, be part of systemic lupus erythematosus, and some other connective tissue diseases such as scleroderma. The phenomenon is usually little more than an annoyance, but if it's a problem drugs called "calcium channel blocking agents" can help make it more tolerable.

"Funny" Fingernails

The nail changes of psoriasis have been mentioned.

The nail fold (the ridge of skin along the sides and base of the fingernail) can exhibit "nail-fold vasculitis" in rheumatoid arthritis and sometimes in lupus. At first glance this can look like a hangnail – a tiny brown-black splinter at the edge of the nail. But these are not hangnails, and they tend to occur in crops, with several fingers showing the same thing at the same time. They are probably similar in origin to the rheumatoid nodule, the result of a combination of rheumatoid inflammation in a tiny blood vessel and local pressure. They are harmless, and tend to come and go.

Hip, Leg and Foot
- hip and leg pain
- kneecap aching (patello-femoral syndrome)
- knee lumps and swellings
- calf pain and/or swelling
- heel pain
- foot numbness
- pain in the ball of the foot

Hip and Leg Pain

Pain from the Lower Back and Sacroiliac Joints
This is often "referred" to the buttock and the back of the upper thigh. It's not sciatic pain, and doesn't mean that there is nerve pressure. This type of referred pain is often described as "dull" or "stiff," and lacks the severity of true sciatica. This location is typical for both ordinary mechanical low back pain and the pain of inflammation, as in ankylosing spondylitis.

If the pain continues below the back of the knee into the calf, sciatica is a distinct possibility. Pain here is caused by pressure on the root of one of the nerves as it leaves the spinal canal to pass down the leg. Sciatic pain is usually not "deep and dull," but sharp and severe. It's often worse with coughing or straining to have a bowel movement and is usually, but not always, made better by lying down.

Pain similar in location – down the back of the thigh and calf – but less intense, and coming on with prolonged standing or walking, is characteristic of "spinal stenosis" (see the section "Low Back Pain").

Pain from Problems in Blood Supply

Another significant leg pain is the pain of peripheral vascular disease or "hardening of the arteries." If the main blood vessels into the legs become narrowed by cholesterol deposits, pain may be the first symptom. It's usually felt in the calf. The patient experiences a severe cramp that causes him or her to sit and rest, and after a minute or two the walk can be resumed. (This kind of pain is called "claudication," after the Roman emperor Claudius, although his leg pain wasn't due to bad circulation.)

Pain from Irritation of the Trochanteric Bursa

On the side of the hip, right where we experience the maximum pressure when we lie on our side in bed, is a bony bump called the "greater trochanter." Because this is a pressure point, like the elbow, there is a bursa over this bump, and it can become very tender. Overlying this bursa is a tough sheet of tissue that covers the outside of the thigh muscle from the pelvis to the knee. This is called the "lateral band" (or iliotibial band) and in middle age it can become very tight and tender, particularly where it passes over the trochanter.

Tenderness in these two structures – bursa and lateral band – is common. Trochanteric bursitis also causes a lot of unnecessary worry. Most people interpret pain here as coming from the hip joint, which it decidedly is not.

Reassurance, stretching exercises and often a local injection of a mixture of corticosteroid and anesthetic usually settle things down.

Pain from the Hip Joint

This is usually felt in the groin, spreading down the front of the thigh toward the knee. Some patients have pain only in the knee area, and it isn't until the doctor tries to move their hips that the true source is discovered. True hip pain is very rarely felt on the side of the hip or deep in the buttock.

Thigh Numbness

Burning numbness of the upper thigh, overlapping the front and side, is due to pressure on a small nerve, the lateral femoral cutaneous nerve, usually just where it enters the leg at the outer groin. It is seen in association with pregnancy, obesity and hernia repair surgery.

Kneecap Aching (Patello-femoral Syndrome)

Kneecap pain is typically described as "deep and aching" and is felt over the front (or front and inner) aspect of the kneecap. It's made worse by going up or down stairs. Sitting in one position for some time is difficult. Women seem to have this symptom more than men, either in their teens or in later middle age. Very often the patient can feel a fine "grating" by cupping the kneecap with the palm of the hand while bending and straightening the knee. Hamstring muscle stretching, strengthening of the quadriceps muscle at the front of the thigh and sometimes taping the kneecap are the usual treatments. Time, and avoidance of things that make the pain worse, helps too.

Knee Lumps and Swellings

There are a number of bursae around the knee, but the one that most commonly "blows up" is the pre-patellar bursa. This condition is called "housemaid's knee," because of the traditional cause – kneeling. However, those I've seen in the past few years have been due to infection more likely than local trauma.

Occasionally other knee region bursae will swell. Swelling just below the kneecap is called "jumper's knee," and a very common one at the back of the knee is discussed below.

The other cause of swelling just below the kneecap is inflammation of the site where the tendon from the kneecap attaches to the shin. This site of attachment is called the tibial tubercle, and it can be felt as a bony bump. Inflammation here, like "jumper's knee," is most often a problem in young male athletes. It's called Osgoode-Schlatter's disease, and it gets better.

Calf Pain and/or Swelling

This symptom, which may come on very suddenly and look just like phlebitis in the calf, is actually due to arthritis in the knee. Behind the knee is a small fluid-filled sac called a "popliteal bursa" or "Baker's cyst." Normally it's very small and inapparent, but if the knee becomes inflamed and swells, the fluid from the swelling can leak backward and swell up the sac. If this happens slowly, over several days to weeks (which is the usual case), the main symptom is usually a sensation of fullness behind the knee, as if a ping-pong ball has been placed there.

Baker's cyst

Buildup of fluid in the knee can cause a Baker's cyst, a swelling behind the knee.

But if the cyst fills up rapidly, its wall can be stretched thin and it can get very large like a balloon. With nowhere to go, it works its way down into the calf, where it can cause quite a bit of pain, particularly if the balloon breaks.

Treatment is directed toward the cause by injecting the knee with cortisone, which takes down the knee inflammation, and the cyst deflates.

Heel Pain

A few years ago, on the first day of a hiking holiday, I awoke and attempted to stand. The moment my left heel made contact with the floor I felt an excruciating pain. I went hiking anyway, but my heel didn't touch the ground at any time. It was a dumb thing to do. The next day my heel was better but my calf was unbearable.

That was my one brief brush with plantar fasciitis. Pain here is usually caused by some form of overuse. The other setting in which it's common is the seronegative forms of spondylarthritis, such as ankylosing spondylitis. Treatment may be a problem, with pain persisting despite NSAIDs and proper insole padding. On occasion I have resorted to local cortisone injections. A special splint can be made, designed to stretch the tight tissues on the sole of the foot while the patient sleeps, but it's expensive.

The other site of pain is at the back of the heel, where the Achilles tendon attaches. Irritation here can be caused by overuse, tight tissues or inflammation. This is one tendon that I would never inject with corticosteroid. It carries enormous loads, and if the injection were to weaken the tendon it would be more likely to rupture than any other tendon in the body.

Foot Numbness

Not too commonly, the small nerves of the foot will become "trapped" at the ankle or between the bones at the ball of the foot. If symptoms of numbness or burning are severe, surgical release of the tissues pressing on the nerves is possible. There are two other causes of foot numbness. Nerve pressure from higher up, often linked to sciatica, is one. The other is a "sensory neuropathy," where the smaller nerves that carry feelings of pressure and pain (from the skin to the spinal cord) are damaged. This can be caused by diabetes and RA, but because there are so many different possibilities a full investigation is usually wise. Typically, the numbness is felt in the foot and ankle in a "stocking" distribution.

Pain in the Ball of the Foot

Pain under the ball of the foot, where the toes attach, is called metatarsalgia. The "ball," the thickened ridge running the width of the forefoot, is formed by the MTP joints (the joints that allow us to wiggle our toes) with a thick layer of padding (mostly fatty tissue) between the joint and the skin.

Metatarsalgia is common, sometimes as a result of the thinning of the fat pad that often comes with age, but more often as a result of inflammatory arthritis, particularly RA. Inflammation here is painful, and damages the joints. This is often linked to the big toe twisting over, causing the second toe to ride up. The deformity at the base of the big toe is called a "bunion."

The result, often, is toes that overlap or toes that ride up – so-called "cock-up" or "hammer" toes. These deformities are due to a combination of inflammation, body weight and constricting footwear. Treatment should include suppressing inflammation, but because a 100 percent result is not always possible, the role of footwear should be considered.

"Walking shoes," built along the lines of the modern running shoe, are great. They have a neutral heel, sharing weight evenly between front and back, and provide excellent ankle and instep support. At least one brand (New Balance) comes in variable widths, which helps to keep the toes from being squashed together. They are well padded, and all have lots of room for the occupational therapist to make an insole to shift the weight off the MTPs.

Common changes in the foot in RA

In rheumatoid arthritis, the weight-bearing soft tissue cushion of the foot commonly migrates forward and the toe slips upward.

Back

- sudden back pain
- night pain

Sudden Back Pain

Sudden back pain is never good news. Usually it's simply an attack of "acute mechanical low back pain" and will be better in a few days to weeks, but it can be quite incapacitating until it is.

If the pain is higher than the "low back" (what people refer to as "the small of the back"), particularly up between the shoulder blades, a compression fracture is a possibility. There are several causes of compression fractures including infection and malignancy, but osteoporosis is high on the list.

Pain coming from deep in the belly – from the stomach, kidney or pancreas, or even the main blood vessel, the aorta – can be felt in the back. Because there are so many possible sources, some of them serious, sudden back pain requires a full assessment by a competent doctor without delay.

Night Pain

Night pain is also, in general, never good news. Ordinary back pain gets better with rest. Night back pain may be due to inflammation, as in ankylosing spondylitis, but it's also a symptom of bone infection and bone tumors, both benign and malignant. Night pain too requires a very careful look by a doctor.

Skin

Bruises and "Hickeys"

Bruising of the skin is not a common problem in arthritis except where an older patient has been taking prednisone for some time. Here, bruises appear suddenly, particularly on the arms, without any known injury. The skin is often paper-thin, and easily torn. Prednisone, even in relatively small doses, causes thinning of the cushion of fat under the skin of the arms. The skin naturally thins with aging, and corticosteroids increase this tendency. These changes all combine to predispose to skin tearing and bruising.

Bruises can also be a problem if the platelets, those blood cells very important in clotting, are reduced in numbers. This can arise as a result of disease, such as lupus, or as a side effect of treatment. Quite a number of drugs can do this.

Clusters of pinpoint bleeding (a "hickey") can result from either disease or drugs. These are most frequent on the shins and should be brought to the doctor's attention.

Joint with Unbearable Pain

Infections love joints that have already been damaged. This is true in OA, in all types of chronic arthritis and in RA. Joint infection is rare, but it's serious.

Infection usually settles in a single joint, at least at first. The pain from the infection is different and much worse than the usual pain of OA or RA. It keeps you awake at night, and brings tears when the joint is moved. Fever or chills may be clues to the true nature of the problem, but may not appear at first. Pain like this demands that a needle be inserted into the joint and a specimen of fluid sent to the lab. Early treatment is essential. Not only can the joint be badly damaged; a delay in diagnosis may result in death.

SEVEN

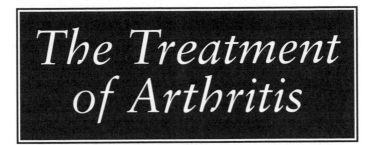

The Treatment of Arthritis

ASA and Its Cousins – the NSAIDs

For a long time, ASA (acetylsalicylic acid, or aspirin) was the only NSAID we had. The first modern NSAIDs were developed in the 1950s and 1960s, and in the last 20 years the number available has grown incredibly; we now have ibuprofen, salsalate, diclofenac, naproxen, ketoprofen, piroxicam, indomethacin, sulindac and others. In the recent past, a new generation of NSAIDs – the COX-2 specific drugs – has been developed. These drugs differ from each other in a number of ways – chemically, how often they need to be taken each day, cost, side effects – but they are very similar in one way: *they all seem to be equally effective as anti-inflammatories.* None of the newer NSAIDs has been shown to be superior to any other, or to ASA itself, in treating the two most common problems, osteoarthritis and rheumatoid arthritis.

NSAIDs are the most commonly prescribed of all drugs in arthritis. Global sales, to an estimated 30 million people, exceed $2 billion (U.S.) each year. Most of these prescriptions are likely inappropriate. Patients and their doctors have been oversold on their supposed benefits. This is particularly true in older people. A 1991 study from the

---

How to Swallow a Pill

Patients with some types of arthritis, as well as older people, may have problems getting a pill from mouth to stomach. The muscle of the swallowing tube, the esophagus, is often weak or uncoordinated. This means that the medication may, though the swallower doesn't know it, get stuck on the way down. This can happen to people with normal swallowing too, especially with big pills. A pill that gets stuck may be very irritating to the lining of the esophagus. Prolonged contact there can cause ulceration, bleeding and, in the long term, scarring.

To reduce the risk of pill injury to the esophagus:
* if possible, get smaller pills, since big ones are more likely to get stuck
* swallow in the upright position, and don't lie down right after taking the pill
* take plenty of water – at least half a glass
* if the pill is big, check with your pharmacist to see if it can be ground up and mixed with a semi-liquid like applesauce

---

province of Alberta found that 26 percent of all those 65 and older had been given a prescription for at least one NSAID over the previous six months. A British study showed the same thing.

However, when prescribed appropriately, NSAIDs are useful because they have a dual action: they are anti-inflammatory, helping to suppress joint swelling, warmth and pain; and they are analgesic, with painkilling properties separate from their anti-inflammatory action.

The following can be said about NSAIDs:

* their effectiveness varies with the kind of arthritis being treated
* they are rarely enough by themselves
* serious complications are uncommon, but can arise without warning
* different patients, even with the same problem, respond differently to the same NSAID

COX-1 and COX-2: What's the Difference?

There was long thought to be just one kind of cyclooxygenase (COX). COX is an enzyme found in many body tissues; it is important in the manufacture of prostaglandins. Prostaglandins are known to be one of the major players in inflammation, and NSAIDs are thought to work because they block COX, and hence the synthesis of prostaglandins. Unfortunately, prostaglandins also have very important roles – such as protecting the stomach against acid damage and ensuring that kidney blood flow is maintained. Up until recently we've had to take the bad with the good; effective NSAID blocking of inflammation often brought with it stomach ulcers and kidney impairment.

We now know there are two kinds of COX. COX-1 makes the "good" prostaglandins, and COX-2 makes the "bad" (inflammatory) ones. All the traditional NSAIDs block the actions of both. Now, however, we have "COX-2 specific" NSAIDs, designed to leave COX-1 alone. Celecoxib and rofecoxib are two of these, and studies have shown that they are associated with a dramatic reduction in stomach ulcer rates. It's important to realize that ulcers may happen for other reasons; while these drugs clearly don't cause stomach ulcers, they may delay the healing of an existing one.

Doctors are also excited about some anti-cancer possibilities of the COX-2 drugs. Both bowel and bladder cancer tissues contain COX-2. Drugs that inhibit this enzyme may inhibit the development of such cancers. It has long been known that ASA use is associated with a lower risk of bowel cancer.

There are some drawbacks, though. Besides the greater cost, it is likely that COX-2 inhibiting drugs still affect kidney blood flow (ankle and foot swelling due to fluid retention is a common side effect). And celecoxib can't be taken by people allergic to sulfa drugs.

Choosing an NSAID

For the individual patient one NSAID often appears to be best. To find that one, a sequence of NSAIDs is prescribed for relatively brief trial periods of about 7 to 10 days each. By the time three or possibly four have been tried, the doctor has a pretty good idea of how much that patient is going to be helped by an NSAID, and which one is best. Trying more would waste time and money.

Ideally, the NSAID chosen will be cheap, well tolerated, easy to remember to take and effective. Few drugs meet all these criteria. The decision is also influenced by whether or not a patient has a drug plan to help with the cost, because some are quite expensive.

You can bleed on any of the traditional NSAIDs, particularly if:

- you are older (the risk increases with age)
- you have had an ulcer before
- you are taking high doses of one NSAID, or combining two
- you are also taking a corticosteroid such as prednisone
- you are on blood-thinning drugs
- you have a serious medical condition;

and, although this is less certain, if

- you smoke cigarettes
- you drink alcohol

Choosing the right NSAID depends on a number of factors. Some are clearly more risky than others. People with a previous ulcer should probably be prescribed either ulcer protection (with misoprostol combined with an NSAID in a single pill, or omeprazole added to an NSAID) or one of the newer COX-2 specific agents. Older people and those on anticoagulant drugs should be treated similarly. And people with borderline kidney or heart function should probably not take any type of NSAID.

One consideration that may have been exaggerated is convenience. Some NSAIDs need to be taken four times daily, others twice daily and a small number once daily. For most patients this is not important, but for others, especially if they're likely to forget a midday dose at work, it very definitely is.

The choice of the NSAIDs tried, and the order in which they are tried, is influenced by their safety profiles. More on that later.

Just How Good Are NSAIDs in Arthritis?

Not as good as we would like. In the most common types of arthritis – rheumatoid arthritis (RA) and osteoarthritis (OA) – NSAIDs are certainly useful, but by themselves they are woefully inadequate.

In RA common practice is to find the best NSAID and then decide on a second-line drug to be *added*. It is seldom that the disease is so mild as to be controlled by NSAIDs alone.

In OA there may be an inflammatory component that is helped by an NSAID, but the chief benefit seems to be pain control. Studies have shown that in osteoarthritis, a simple analgesic like acetaminophen is often just as good as an NSAID, and safer and cheaper.

In some diseases NSAIDs are very effective: in crystal arthritis, such as gout, NSAID response is spectacular – unless treatment is started too late, or the dose is inadequate. In ankylosing spondylitis, an NSAID usually results in the patient's first good night of sleep in years.

Side Effects of the Older NSAIDs

Rare Side Effects
- skin rash, including photosensitivity (a rash provoked by going out in the sun) and hives
- jaundice or other evidence of liver problems
- bowel ulceration and bleeding
- impaired production of blood cells (aplastic anemia)
- asthma
- significant kidney impairment
- confusion, headache and neck stiffness

Common Side Effects
- indigestion
- stomach ulceration and bleeding

Some of the rarer side effects are linked to specific NSAIDs (such as aplastic anemia with phenylbutazone), while others may be seen with any NSAID. For example, if an asthma attack is provoked by one NSAID, all (including ASA) should be avoided. In special circumstances, if the NSAID is badly needed, the patient can be desensitized.

All NSAIDs also appear to affect kidney blood flow. This is not a problem for most people, but it's a big problem for:

- older people
- people with kidney function that is already below normal
- people on some other drugs (such as diuretics, given to get rid of excess body fluid or to treat high blood pressure)

These people may be affected quite badly, by worsening kidney function, more fluid retention, worsening blood pressure control and even heart failure.

The common side effects, those affecting the gut, are the real problem. NSAID indigestion is common; about 10 to 20 percent of users will experience it at some time. But it's an unreliable marker for an ulcer, which can bleed without any warning signs. And many with indigestion don't have ulcers.

Taking an NSAID increases the risk of developing an ulcer, having gastrointestinal bleeding or experiencing an ulcer perforation by about five times. The risk of a bleeding ulcer in an otherwise healthy person taking one of the older NSAIDs has been estimated at 1 to 2 for every 100 patient years. In other words, if 100 patients take the NSAID for a year, 1 or 2 of them will develop an ulcer in that year.

Only about half of all ulcers will cause symptoms. Very often the first sign of an ulcer is evidence of bleeding, such as vomiting of blood, black bowel movements or light-headedness and fainting.

There are a number of ulcer-protective drugs available, but only misoprostol and omeprazole have been convincingly shown to reduce the risk.

For indigestion alone, anti-ulcer drugs can be tried. They may or may not clear up the symptom. Since the cause of non-ulcer indigestion isn't known, it can be difficult to deal with. Sometimes it's so bad that the best solution is simply to stop the NSAID.

Other NSAID Issues

Taking an NSAID on an "as needed" basis (a pill or two today, then a few days skipped) is foolish. NSAIDs need several days to develop their full effect, and little can be expected from occasional doses except possibly heartburn or an ulcer. The ulcer doctors see much more ulcer bleeding in occasional NSAID users than they do in patients with arthritis. It's surprising how many people take ASA for stomach aches or insomnia.

Most pharmacists recommend that an NSAID be taken with food. It's doubtful this really helps prevent an ulcer, but meals do help as reminders.

NSAIDs come in suppository form as well as tablets and capsules, but there's no evidence that suppositories cause fewer ulcers.

NSAIDs may interact with other drugs, and can cause real problems:

- with blood-thinning agents (anticoagulants), serious bleeding may result
- with lithium, toxic blood levels of lithium can occur
- with a variety of blood pressure medications, high blood pressure control may worsen. Sulindac may possibly be the safest NSAID in this setting.

Finally, there is nothing magic about an NSAID. If you don't think it's helping, stop taking it. If symptoms of pain or stiffness or even increased joint swelling reappear, you need it and you can restart it. You may have to wait a few days to feel its full effect, but if it was helping before and nothing else has changed, it will work again.

Cortisone – The Adrenocorticosteroids

Adrenocorticosteroids (also called corticosteroids) are the most powerful anti-inflammatory drugs we have. Were it not for their side effects we would use them much more freely. They are essential in the treatment of some forms of arthritis, such as systemic lupus erythematosus and polymyalgia rheumatica, where the decision to use them is taken with full knowledge of the risks involved. They are also widely used, over the short term or in low doses (in which case the risk of side effects is minimized), to supplement the main treatment in several other conditions.

Rheumatoid arthritis is a good example of such a condition, and it was in rheumatoid arthritis that the first corticosteroid, cortisone, was used. In 1949, Dr. Philip Hench of the Mayo Clinic gave it to a number of patients. The effect was spectacular. I've seen the "before and after" movies Hench took of his patients, painfully climbing, and then leaping, over a bench barrier. So impressive was the result that Hench was among the winners of the 1950 Nobel prize in medicine. It was several years before it was realized that this "cure" for rheumatoid arthritis was flawed, and that it carried a price. That price was the syndrome of hypercortisonism.

First, though, a few words of clarification. There are a number of chemical compounds that qualify as "steroids" – Vitamin D and male sex hormones among them – but when the term is used in medicine it almost always refers to cortisol, produced by the adrenal gland, or one of its synthetic cousins. Of these, cortisone and hydrocortisone were the first to be made commercially; nowadays the most commonly used (and cheapest) is prednisone.

Problems with corticosteroids are of two types – those arising from using doses higher than the amount the body normally makes each day (the equivalent of about 7.5 milligrams of prednisone), and those arising from the sudden withdrawal of corticosteroid medication. The likelihood, and severity, of both are directly related to the size of the daily dose and the length of time it is given.

Problems from High, and Prolonged, Corticosteroid Use

Hypercortisonism
When the dose of prednisone (or another similar synthetic corticosteroid) exceeds 7.5 milligrams a day for more than three to four weeks, signs of hypercortisonism begin to develop. Hypercortisonism caused by prednisone is identical to Cushing's syndrome, a disease state where the adrenal glands produce cortisol in excess.

Fully developed, hypercortisonism may include any or all of the following features:

- increased appetite and weight gain, especially on the trunk and face. A chubby face is typical of someone on high-dose, long-term prednisone
- easy bruising and skin fragility of the arms and legs, especially in older people
- cataract development
- mood changes. Mild euphoria is common, but depression may occur. Insomnia is frequent
- high blood pressure
- extra insulin required by diabetics because of higher blood sugars, and "pre-diabetics" becoming overtly diabetic
- stomach ulcers, if the patient is taking NSAIDs at the same time
- stunting of growth in children

Osteonecrosis
"Osteonecrosis" is doctor-talk for dead bone. It is a specific type of dead bone, the kind that results when an area of bone loses its blood supply. If this happens near a joint – and the hip is a favorite target – the area of dead bone may collapse, a catastrophe that inevitably ends up with surgery and a total hip replacement.

Cortisone-like drugs have for a long time been seen as the culprit in osteonecrosis, although this has been hard to prove. Many diseases for which corticosteroids are used – such as lupus and Crohn's disease – may themselves be responsible for osteonecrosis.

Fortunately, osteonecrosis from prednisone is rare. I've never yet had a patient develop it.

Hardening of the Arteries (Atherosclerosis)

There is no question that the long-term use of prednisone in systemic lupus erythematosus increases the risk of hardening of the arteries and, in particular, coronary artery disease. These conditions substantially increase the risk of stroke and heart attack. There is still some debate as to whether or not prednisone has the same effect in rheumatoid arthritis. Antimalarial drugs, such as hydroxychloroquine, have an opposite, protective effect. Since they are also helpful in treating the inflammation of both diseases, this "side effect" is a real bonus and can justify treatment with these two drugs at the same time.

Osteoporosis

Bone is a living tissue. Old bone is continuously being broken down, in patches. This process is followed almost immediately by the laying down of new bone by bone-forming cells. The two processes of breakdown and repair are normally in balance. When the rate of breakdown exceeds repair, bone mass (solidity) is reduced. We call this osteoporosis.

Between 10 and 20 percent of all patients with rheumatoid arthritis, who are on long-term corticosteroids, will experience crush fractures of one or more vertebrae in the backbone. The risk of hip fracture is 50 percent.

Normal versus osteoporotic bone

| Normal | Osteoporotic |

Comparison of normal bone and osteoporotic bone. The figure on the left shows a cross-section of a normal vertebra; the figure on the right demonstrates the effects of osteoporotic depletion.

This risk of fracture can be estimated in any patient, on corticosteroids or not, by measuring bone mineral density (through a technique known as DEXA – dual energy X-ray absorptiometry). Ordinary X-rays won't do; up to half of bone mass must be lost before they will detect the change.

How Does Osteoporosis Come About?
Bone breakdown continues at a constant rate throughout life. The rate of bone repair, however, slows down in older people. It also slows in those who are physically inactive, in post-menopausal women with the drop in estrogen production, and in those who get inadequate supplies of calcium and vitamin D. Often, many of these factors are combined.

Corticosteroids magnify problems in bone repair. They can cause osteoporosis in anyone, young or old, but the effect is most obvious in post-menopausal women (who already exhibit many of the osteoporosis risk factors). They do this quite quickly, particularly within the first 6 to 12 months of treatment. Corticosteroids affect several key ele-

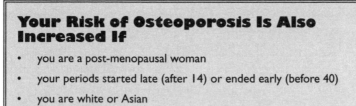

Your Risk of Osteoporosis Is Also Increased If

- you are a post-menopausal woman
- your periods started late (after 14) or ended early (before 40)
- you are white or Asian
- you are housebound and elderly
- you weigh less than 120 pounds (55 kg)
- you smoke cigarettes

ments in bone repair. The amount of calcium available for new bone formation is reduced. They both slow dietary calcium absorption in the intestine and speed its removal from blood by the kidney. They stimulate the bone cells that promote bone breakdown, and inhibit the bone cells that promote bone growth.

What this means is that every patient who is started on prednisone for anything but a very short period must also be started on an anti-osteoporosis program.

- If the patient is a post-menopausal woman, replacement estrogen should be seriously considered. Raloxifene is an alternative to estrogen, although it doesn't help menopausal symptoms like hot flashes. It does resemble estrogen in its beneficial effects on bone, yet – and this is important if there is a fear of uterus or breast cancer – it does not affect the lining of the uterus or breast tissue.
- A regular program of aerobic physical activity should be designed, if necessary with the assistance of a physiotherapist, keeping the problems imposed by the arthritis in mind.
- A daily calcium intake of at least 1,000 milligrams should be achieved. One cup of milk will provide 300 milligrams,

a cup of yogurt about 400 milligrams. Calcium-containing antacid tablets are another inexpensive source.

- A low dose (800 or 900 units) of vitamin D daily is desirable. Vitamin D is essential to normal bone development. People who are elderly or housebound are very often vitamin D deficient, and have a greatly increased risk of fracture.
- If it is likely that prednisone will be needed for more than a few weeks, a bisphosphonate can be used to slow bone breakdown. Etidronate, alendronate and pamidronate are bisphosphonates. They have been proved effective in both the prevention and the treatment of osteoporosis.

Problems from the Sudden Withdrawal of Corticosteroid Medication

When corticosteroids are used in doses of more than the equivalent of 7.5 milligrams of prednisone a day, the adrenal gland does not make cortisol. This is not a problem if drugs like prednisone are used for short periods only. But when such doses are used continuously for prolonged periods (three months is considered the cut-off), cortisol production will be completely suppressed. The patient is now dependent on a source outside the body for corticosteroid.

Since corticosteroids are essential for life, and are particularly important in helping the body deal with major physical stress, their sudden absence – if for any reason the patient stops taking daily prednisone – can have serious consequences. If adrenal gland suppression is only partial, symptoms of fatigue, nausea, loss of appetite and muscle pain may develop. If suppression is total, the patient may experience the life-threatening state doctors call "shock." The only safe way to reduce, and stop, corticosteroids is slowly, over a period of weeks to months. But even if the patient has managed to achieve this, the body may not completely recover its ability to produce large amounts of cortisol in circumstances of stress until a year or more goes by.

Because of this, patients who are on (or have been on) corticosteroids must be given extra corticosteroid if they are exposed to severe physical stress. Such events as an automobile accident or major surgery call for immediate corticosteroid treatment, usually by needle, into a vein.

Patients on corticosteroids should never stop their medication suddenly. If unable to take their regular dose, they should contact a physician. They should also carry a wallet card (or wear a medical-alert bracelet) indicating that they are on a corticosteroid.

To Sum Up

The most effective way to avoid the unwelcome side effects of corticosteroids is not to take them. Regrettably, this is not always possible. Next best is to minimize the damage by attempting to keep the dose as low as possible most of the time, and to keep periods of high-dose treatment short. If at all possible, the daily dose should be taken as a single morning dose, since normal cortisol production is much less likely to be suppressed when this is done. And corticosteroids should never be stopped suddenly if they have been taken continuously for more than a week or two.

"Second-Line" Drugs

The name "second-line" comes from the fact that in rheumatoid arthritis the NSAIDs are used first. When their effect has been determined, assuming there is still a problem, the drugs in this class are then called upon.

We used to call second-line drugs "remitting agents," but it's clear that they don't cause the disease to go away. Some doctors call them DMARDs (Disease-Modifying Anti-Rheumatic Drugs), which they are, and some call them SAARDs (Slow-Acting Anti-Rheumatic Drugs), which they also are.

The two major differences, in practical terms, between these drugs and NSAIDs are that they take much longer to have an effect (usually months), and they are much more effective in suppressing the disease process. Unfortunately, another characteristic of drugs in this category is the fact that they often lose their effect as time goes by.

This means that, after several years, many patients will have acquired experience with quite a number of these agents. Fortunately, research into new drugs in this area has managed to keep pace. The list keeps getting longer, but the main second-line drugs at present are:

- methotrexate
- gold by injection
- azathioprine
- sulfasalazine
- D-penicillamine
- hydroxychloroquine
- oral gold

These drugs are unrelated to each other chemically. Almost all were first used in arthritis for reasons that were later shown to be wrong, or as a result of a series of chance observations.

Gold, for instance, was used because RA was once thought to be caused by tuberculosis, and gold salts have some activity against TB in a test-tube. Methotrexate, when it was first used in psoriasis, was observed to help control psoriatic arthritis so it was used in RA, where it was found to work even better. It is only now, in the age of genetic engineering, that we may be developing a series of "designer drugs" specifically for arthritis.

When Are These Drugs Used?

In rheumatoid arthritis, right away.

This category of drug is introduced early, usually within months of the diagnosis, since we have come to appreciate that effective treatment must not be delayed, that this class of drug is far superior to NSAIDs and that the risk of side effects has been greatly exaggerated. Investigation makes a convincing case that many of these drugs are actually less harmful than NSAIDs!

Unfortunately, these agents are not uniformly effective in all forms of arthritis. They are used primarily in just two forms of inflammatory arthritis: rheumatoid and psoriatic. Some are used as "supportive" treatment in a few other conditions, in particular ankylosing spondylitis, systemic lupus erythematosus, polymyositis and dermatomyositis. There is no "second-line" treatment available for the most common problem of all, osteoarthritis. Nor is there specific treatment for fibromyalgia, chondrocalcinosis, polymyalgia rheumatica, scleroderma or Sjögren's syndrome.

Which One to Choose?

These are my preferred second-line drugs, in order of *safety*:

- hydroxychloroquine
- auranofin – an oral gold compound
- sulfasalazine
- methotrexate
- azathioprine
- sodium aurothiomalate – an intramuscular gold compound
- D-penicillamine
- cyclosporin

Another rheumatologist has a slightly different list, based

on treatment of almost 3,000 patients. His study ranked the following in order of safety:

- hydroxychloroquine
- intramuscular gold
- D-penicillamine, methotrexate and azathioprine (all statistically similar)
- oral gold

When he compared NSAIDs to these agents, several, including indomethacin, tolmetin, ketoprofen and piroxicam, had higher "toxicity profiles" than did hydroxychloroquine and intramuscular gold.

In order of *effectiveness*, my list looks like this:

- methotrexate
- sodium aurothiomalate
- azathioprine
- sulfasalazine
- D-penicillamine
- hydroxychloroquine
- auranofin

Cyclosporin and three very expensive but also very effective newcomers – etanercept, infliximab and leflunomide – may work best when teamed up with methotrexate (see below).

Second-line Drug Combinations

One very exciting development in the past few years has been the discovery that some of the second-line drugs may be more effective in combination than singly. Already I am starting to "double up" when a patient with RA doesn't show early benefit from one drug. Rather than waiting to see what a month or two more will bring (since I am now very aware of the narrow window of opportunity for preventing joint damage), I add a second drug – or even two. I expect that in the near future it will become almost routine to start all RA patients on two or more second-line drugs right at the beginning.

Some promising combinations include

- methotrexate and sulfasalazine and hydroxychloroquine
- methotrexate and cyclosporin
- methotrexate and intramuscular gold
- methotrexate and etanercept
- methotrexate and leflunomide
- methotrexate and infliximab

Etanercept, infliximab and leflunomide are part of the new wave of second-line drugs. The older medications in this category were found to be effective more or less by accident. The new ones are "designer drugs," specifically synthesized to interfere with the various stages of joint inflammation.

Methotrexate (MTX)
This is the drug I prescribe first in RA if there is active inflammation with significant disability. The risk of serious side effects is low. It promises early onset of action, usually within four to six weeks, and the likelihood of a sustained and prolonged effect. MTX is used extensively in psoriatic arthritis, and has also found a place in the treatment of systemic lupus and polymyositis, where it seems to permit the use of lower doses of corticosteroid.

MTX is usually given as tablets, but can also be injected into muscles.

The effective weekly dose for a patient may be as low as two 2.5-milligram tablets, or as high as ten. The average is five tablets (12.5 milligrams) once a week. Because the effective dose range is so wide, it's best to start low (three tablets a week), and only slowly increase the dose by one tablet each time. Changes in dose should occur no more often than every three weeks; once a month is the usual. All the pills should be taken together, at the same time, on the same day each week.

It isn't unusual to notice a good response at a fairly low dose at first, but then to require a higher dose later on to maintain that response.

A complete blood count (hemoglobin, white cell and platelet counts) is usually done every two weeks until the final dose is decided, then every four to six weeks. Liver function tests should be checked at every second blood test.

Side Effects of Methotrexate

Note that impairment of kidney function increases the risk of any of these side effects. NSAIDs don't interact with MTX when MTX is taken in the doses recommended; however, sulfa-containing antibiotics increase the risk of side effects and should be avoided. Side effects are often dealt with by decreasing the dose or temporarily stopping MTX and then restarting it.

Common to Occasional
- a 12- to 24-hour reaction to the weekly dose. Nausea is most common, but some patients report "flushing" or a temporary flare-up of arthritis. These reactions can be blocked by a small dose of a steroid called dexamethasone, taken with MTX. Nausea with vomiting very occasionally occurs.
- mild anemia, and occasionally lower numbers of white blood cells or platelets, though not low enough to cause problems

- small sores inside the mouth for a day or two after the weekly dose. Both these and anemia (above) can be helped by a low dose of folic acid daily. Note that a high dose of folic acid will counteract the good effects of the MTX.
- a small amount of hair loss, noticeable on the pillow each morning but not obvious to friends and neighbors
- temporary reduction in the sperm count in men may be caused by MTX. In women, MTX should be avoided in pregnancy (it can cause a miscarriage) and breast-feeding.

Rare (If You Suspect One of These, Stop MTX and Call Your Doctor)
- significant lowering of blood counts (hemoglobin, white blood cells, platelets) with symptoms of tiredness, dizziness, infection, bruising or bleeding
- cramps and diarrhea
- "allergic pneumonia" – fever, cough that doesn't bring up anything, shortness of breath
- infection, including pneumonia and shingles
- skin rash (very uncommon). Occasionally, patients with RA who have rheumatoid nodules will develop many new ones, even though the arthritis is under good control.

Very Rare
- liver damage. To be on the safe side, no use of alcohol (except at weddings, birthdays and Christmas), since alcohol may combine with MTX to damage the liver. Psoriasis, obesity and possibly diabetes may also increase the risk of MTX liver damage.

Possible but Not Proved
- increased risk of infection after joint surgery
- a very few cases of lymphoma (a type of lymph gland

cancer) have been discovered in patients treated with MTX (see below under "Azathioprine"). These resolved when MTX was stopped.

Sodium Aurothiomalate (Gold by Injection)

Intramuscular gold is the traditional #1 drug in RA, with over 50 years of clinical use. There is little risk of an unanticipated surprise with gold, and it has a reasonably sustained effect over the long term. The major disadvantages include the need to visit the doctor each week, and the long time it may take to begin to work (12 to 20 weeks).

To make sure the patient isn't sensitive to gold, two small test doses of aurothiomalate are given, one week apart. After that, the regular dose (50 milligrams) is given once a week. The practice in the past was to do this, once a week, until 1,000 milligrams had been given, and some doctors still do this. If the patient is no better, they then try another drug. The problem is that some patients may show a great deal of improvement long before five months (the time needed to give 1,000 milligrams) are up and others will need quite a bit longer.

Most rheumatologists will start to space the doses out, at first to every second week, and then to every third, when they feel the maximum benefit has been reached. It's possible, but unusual, to be able to space the doses out to once a month. Once a patient is on a "maintenance schedule," it is continued indefinitely (for years), even if the arthritis seems to have disappeared. If the arthritis flares up (it very often does), it is important to realize that the gold hasn't lost its effect. It simply needs to be given more often.

Because the blood and urine side effects may turn up at any time, the patient should have a blood and urine test each time an injection is given, although if the patient has been safely on gold for several years, this is sometimes spaced out to every second injection.

Side Effects of Gold Injections

Common to Occasional
- sore mouth and itchy skin, often the first sign of side effects. If gold is continued on the same schedule, mouth ulceration and more extensive skin rash may result. The dose should be withheld for a week or two, until the symptoms subside. Injections can then be resumed, either with a reduced dose or with an increased interval between shots.

Rare
- flare-up of arthritis symptoms, or facial "flushing" and headache, following the weekly injection. This is often controlled by the use of prednisone, given only on the day of the injection. There is no risk of steroid side effects with this.
- thrombocytopenia (a drop in the level of platelets in the blood). If this level falls below a certain point, there is a risk of bruising or even uncontrolled bleeding. The drop is due to an allergic reaction to the gold, and most often reverses if the drug is stopped. Sometimes steroids are used to treat the allergic reaction and speed recovery.
- proteinuria (the "leakage" of a protein [albumin] into the urine in abnormally high amounts). Normally the kidney filter is very fine, but an allergic reaction to gold may cause the kidney "pores" to enlarge and allow the large albumin molecules to escape. Proteinuria is very much like thrombocytopenia. It clears up when gold is stopped, but this may take some time and may require corticosteroids.

Very Rare
- a drop in the white blood cell count, or aplastic anemia (where the bone marrow stops production of red and white blood cells, as well as platelets). These complications may be fatal.
- colitis, with severe diarrhea
- hepatitis
- gold "pneumonia"
- severe generalized skin rash

Azathioprine

Over the last few years I have found myself using more and more of this agent for RA, primarily in instances where methotrexate and gold have failed. It is also used for systemic lupus and in some patients with psoriatic arthritis. It's a fairly safe and effective drug that usually begins to give relief after two to three months, and continues to work moderately well over the long term.

Azathioprine is taken daily. The initial dose is one tablet (50 milligrams), and the dose is later adjusted according to the patient's weight. Later, if the patient has done well, the dose can often be reduced without losing the effect. Once a regular dose has been settled on, complete blood counts (CBC) and liver tests are needed less frequently than with methotrexate and gold, but still should be checked at least every three months.

Side Effects of Azathioprine

Common to Occasional
- mild nausea
- fatigue
- fever

Rare
- hepatitis, with fever, skin rash and liver-enzyme abnormalities
- low hemoglobin, low white blood cell count (and possible infection)
- skin rash

Very Rare or Possible but Not Proved
- malignant lymphoma. Experience in kidney transplant patients has led to concern, and long-standing debate, as to whether azathioprine can cause this type of lymph gland cancer in rheumatoid arthritics.

Even without azathioprine, the risk of lymphoma for patients with RA is increased slightly over the risk in the general population. One study has suggested that azathioprine doubles this extremely small risk. On the other hand, a long-term British study of patients receiving azathioprine for inflammatory bowel disease failed to demonstrate any increase in cancer risk. There were no patients with lymphoma reported.

Sulfasalazine
North American experience with this drug in the treatment of RA has been limited, but since it's a mainstay in the treatment of inflammatory bowel disease, its side effects are well known. The British seem to be quite enthusiastic, and to rank it somewhere near intramuscular gold. Its safety profile is very encouraging, it's fairly effective, and it takes action in two to three months. Its benefits are sustained moderately well over the long term.

There are conflicting reports as to whether sulfasalazine is useful in some of the seronegative arthritis conditions, particularly psoriatic arthritis and ankylosing spondylitis.

Sulfasalazine should be started with a low dose and gradually built up. Start with one tablet (500 milligrams) a day for a week, then increase the daily dose by one tablet each week until, by the fourth week, the patient is taking two tablets twice a day. Occasionally the dose is increased to three tablets twice a day. Once a final dose has been settled on, complete blood counts (CBC) and liver tests are done monthly.

Side Effects of Sulfasalazine
Warning – this drug contains sulfa and should not be taken if you are allergic to sulfa drugs.

Common to Occasional
- nausea or vague abdominal "unease"
- loss of appetite
- "dizziness," headache
- temporary lowering of the sperm count in men (reversible when the drug is stopped)
- yellowish-orange discoloration of the urine

Rare
- skin rash, which may be quite extensive and severe

Very Rare
- severe drop in white blood cell count and platelet count, with infection and bleeding possible
- allergic hepatitis
- allergic pneumonia

D-penicillamine
The dose of this drug has to be built up very slowly to avoid very serious (though rare) side effects. Nevertheless, when other drugs fail, D-penicillamine may be used as it helps many.

It begins to give relief within three to six months, and the effects continue moderately well over the long term.

It's important to start with a low daily dose of D-penicillamine (no more than 250 milligrams), and only slowly increase the daily dose (125 to 250 milligrams each time, no more often than every eight weeks). The maximum daily dose should not exceed 1,000 milligrams. D-penicillamine should be taken on an empty stomach, no closer to a meal than one hour, or it won't all be absorbed into the body.

Despite its name, this drug does not cross-react with penicillin. People with penicillin allergy may take it in safety.

Side Effects of D-penicillamine

Common to Occasional
- mild nausea, metallic taste in the mouth
- minor skin rash, sores in mouth
- small amounts of protein in urine

Rare
- drop in platelet count (with risk of bleeding)
- large amounts of protein in urine (see under "Gold by Injection")

Very Rare
- can cause illnesses that look like dermatomyositis, systemic lupus or myasthenia gravis (a condition of severe muscle weakness)
- major drop in red cell, white blood cell count

Hydroxychloroquine
Hydroxychloroquine is a drug originally developed for use against malaria, but it has been found to be very helpful in

several kinds of arthritis. It's considered to be much weaker than almost all the other "slow-acting drugs." Its safety profile, however, is so good that in a patient with relatively mild RA it's a good choice. It takes effect in three to six months, but its long-term benefit in RA is not as good as that of other drugs.

It's also used in systemic lupus erythematosus, particularly if skin, joint and muscle symptoms are prominent. It appears to counteract the lipid (blood-fat) elevating effect of the corticosteroids that are often used in these same patients. Occasionally it's very helpful in psoriatic arthritis, although in a few patients the psoriasis will worsen significantly.

It's very important, if the risk of eye damage (see section on side effects) is to be avoided, that, in addition to annual eye checks, the dose is carefully calculated, based on the patient's "ideal" body weight. The maximum daily dose is 400 milligrams of hydroxychloroquine (200 milligrams twice a day), but that is for anyone over 130 pounds (59 kg). Those who weigh less must take less. A 110 pounder (50 kg) should get 300 milligrams daily. Using these precautions, I have never seen or heard of a patient developing eye damage.

Side Effects of Hydroxychloroquine

Common to Occasional
- nausea, mild abdominal discomfort

Rare
- skin rash
- muscle weakness
- dizziness

Very Rare
- permanent damage to the retina of the eye, leading to blindness. Fewer than a dozen cases of this have been reported in the world medical literature in patients for whom hydroxychloroquine (as opposed to the older drug chloroquine) was used, where kidney function was normal and the dose was based on body weight. Nonetheless, an annual eye check is prudent.

Auranofin

Oral gold has proved to be a disappointment. Initially it was hoped it would be as effective as intramuscular gold. However, it isn't, and with its annoying tendency to cause diarrhea it has slipped to last place on most physicians' lists. It has a good safety record but doesn't take effect until after three to four months, and the long-term benefits are below average.

There is very little flexibility in the dose of auranofin – one 3 milligram tablet twice a day. A complete blood count (CBC) and urinalysis should be done monthly.

Side Effects of Auranofin

Common to Occasional
- abdominal discomfort, loose stools, diarrhea
- skin rash

Very Rare
- protein in urine, lowered blood count

Cyclosporin

Introduced as a means of blocking the rejection of organ transplants (such as kidney grafts), this powerful immunosuppressive has been shown to be quite effective in RA. There are some real advantages in combining it with methotrexate. The effect may be better than the effect of either drug used alone, and a lower dose of cyclosporin can be used. A lower dose reduces the risk of side effects.

I don't use the combination often; I usually reserve it for cases in which methotrexate in full doses has failed to put out the fire and I am very concerned that joint damage will occur in the immediate future.

The daily dose is calculated on ideal body weight. It can be taken with food, but never with grapefruit juice, which can increase the amount of drug your body absorbs and lead to side effects. A number of drugs can also affect the level of cyclosporin in your body: some antibiotics, antifungal agents, anticonvulsants and even some heart and blood pressure medicines. Check with your pharmacist if you are on any of these.

Because cyclosporin can cause high blood pressure and affect kidney function, blood pressure and kidney blood tests should be checked carefully before treatment and every two weeks for the first three months, then once a month.

Side Effects of Cyclosporin
- rise in serum creatinine (indicating reduced kidney function)
- elevated blood pressure
- headache
- nausea
- increase in body hair
- fluid retention (ankle swelling)
- hand tremor (shakiness)

Depending on the nature of the side effect, I either reduce the daily dose or stop the cyclosporin entirely. Fortunately, this has been necessary in only a few of my patients.

There is no convincing evidence that cyclosporin increases the risk of infection or cancer. However, it should not be used if there is an existing cancer or infection, just as it should not be used in people with abnormal kidney function or uncontrolled high blood pressure.

Etanercept, Infliximab, Leflunomide

These are the new kids on the block. They were specifically designed to affect rheumatoid inflammation.

Inflammation in RA is a very complex process. We believe it starts when one of the class of cells that guards the body against foreign invaders (in ordinary inflammation these are usually bacteria or viruses) comes into contact with something that triggers the alarm. One form the alarm takes is a whole battery of chemical messengers, called cytokines, that are released into the joint. These recruit other cells, the white blood cells that produce antibodies and the white blood cells that attack and kill other cells and bacteria. One form this killing takes is the release into the immediate area of very "corrosive" chemicals. Joint tissue, an innocent bystander, is damaged. Furthermore, cytokines stimulate the lining of the joint to grow and produce other chemicals that break down cartilage. Cytokines are released into the blood stream, and cause fever and fatigue. Finally, because the body is so finely balanced, there are also cytokines released that tend to damp down the inflammation. Unfortunately, in the RA joint these "good" cytokines tend to become overwhelmed by the "bad" or pro-inflammatory cytokines.

One of the key cytokines that promotes inflammation is a substance called TNF-alpha. Produced by both the "guard" cells (macrophages) and the joint-lining tissues, it is released into the surrounding tissues, joint fluid and blood. It stimulates other white blood cells to expand the inflammatory reaction. To do this it must attach itself to the other cells at a specific binding site – like a key in a lock.

Etanercept and *infliximab* have been designed to interfere with this stimulatory action of TNF-alpha. *Etanercept* does this very cleverly; it's a molecule that looks exactly like the keyhole. As long as there is enough of it in circulation (it has to be self-injected twice weekly under the skin), it will prevent enough keys from finding the lock they were intended for, and the inflammation will be damped down.

Infliximab has a similar effect, but it consists of an antibody (a protein specifically designed to attach to another protein) against TNF-alpha. Once the key has an antibody stuck to it, it no longer fits the lock. Infliximab too has to be given by needle – in this case into a vein – but fortunately only once every two months.

Leflunomide is different. It doesn't block TNF-alpha, but it does interfere with the normal functioning of one of the key cells (the lymphocyte) affected by TNF-alpha, and thus interferes with the development of joint inflammation.

Both etanercept and infliximab appear to be remarkably safe, although they do come with a warning to stop using them temporarily if an infection occurs. The worry is that they may be effective enough to interfere with the body's own inflammatory reaction to the infection. Doctors are also concerned that there may be an increase in the cancer rate in the long run. However, so far this hasn't happened.

The big drawback of these new treatments is their price – considerably more than the older standbys. My feeling is that if they prevent joint damage and disability, they will pay for themselves many times over. I expect that in a few years most people with RA will be given a reasonable but short time on methotrexate, and if they don't improve one of these newcomers will be added.

Minocycline

A popular North American radio doctor has for several years pushed the use of tetracycline-group antibiotics for just about every kind of arthritis and muscle ache and pain. His reasoning is that there are all sorts of infectious organisms in people, and that infectious organisms have been shown to trigger certain kinds of arthritis. Besides, he reasons, tetracycline-group antibiotics – including minocycline and doxycycline – can't hurt. So, many of my patients ask me for antibiotics for their arthritis. I tell them that:

- life is a lot more complicated than that. While infection may play a role in some kinds of arthritis, it has not been proven in most. It is a very old idea – sixty years ago, doctors recommended that RA patients undergo total dental extraction and sinus drainage surgery on the theory that RA was caused by chronic infection
- minocycline does more than kill bugs. It also interferes with the release of a chemical (nitric oxide) that kills cartilage cells, and with enzymes that break down cartilage. It may do other good things, like interfere with inflammation and immune reactions
- research has shown that minocycline, taken for several months, is helpful – especially in mild, early RA. I think it is about as effective as hydroxychloroquine or auranofin. I certainly would not recommend it as a single, first-choice drug to anyone with aggressive RA
- minocycline may be worth a try in combination with another second-line drug – when methotrexate has been helpful, for instance, but there is still a fair amount of inflammation

Side Effects of Minocycline

Most side effects are mild – although dizziness, nausea and headache may cause up to a quarter of patients to abandon the drug. There have also been a very few instances when, used to treat acne, minocycline caused systemic lupus (SLE) and autoimmune hepatitis. And hyperpigmentation of the skin or gums – blue-gray discoloration either diffusely in the skin and gums, or locally, in old skin scars – is fairly common. Both types gradually fade when minocycline is stopped.

Physiotherapy, Occupational Therapy and Social Work

The following illustrates how my community's arthritis treatment team works.

Debbie is a 33-year-old primary school teacher. She and her husband Mike have been married for three years.

Debbie came to me because of progressive joint pain and swelling over the past year. Despite her pain, and the severe fatigue that accompanied it, I sensed that she probably wouldn't have come if she weren't having trouble coping at work – she'd been forced to take a total of ten sick days over the past four months.

My diagnosis was rheumatoid arthritis and, after an initial period of NSAID treatment alone, I started Debbie on methotrexate and low-dose prednisone.

Debbie was obviously relieved that I could put a label on her problem. She had been concerned that her symptoms were "all in her head," and suspected that Mike thought so too. This relief, though, was short-lived. She began to push herself harder. She took on extra responsibilities at school and spent her weekends trying to ensure that her home was immaculate. She tried to deal with her illness by denying its existence.

This phase didn't last. On a visit a month or two after the diagnosis had been made, she broke into tears. She confessed that she wasn't sleeping and had difficulty concentrating. She was depressed.

I realized that both Debbie and I needed help. I asked her if she would like to see our arthritis team's social worker. I explained that she could only benefit from an exploration of her emotional reactions to her arthritis. I also thought the social worker could help her develop more constructive strategies to deal with the realities of chronic illness. Debbie agreed, and I made the referral. And realizing that in my focus on controlling her arthritis with drugs I had ignored other equally important aspects of treatment, I requested both a physiotherapy and occupational therapy consultation.

The Social Worker Comments:

During our first session, I explained to Debbie that she would have an opportunity to explore the impact arthritis had on her personally, on her relationships, and on her place in the community. We agreed to meet for several sessions to do some problem-solving in the areas Debbie identified as stressors.

Individual Intervention

Debbie confessed that her self-esteem had taken a beating. It had always been linked to her ability to demonstrate, to herself and to others, that she could take on a challenge. Her sense of worth, being tied to her productivity, had nose-dived.

In our discussions, Debbie came to realize that the message she received as she was growing up was "the harder you work, the better," and that this was now working against her. She came to recognize that self-worth does not depend on accomplishments. What were important were her unique qualities as a person, her personality, her strengths and skills, and these arthritis could never take away from her.

She began to practice "self-talk." When a negative message, such as "I feel useless since I can't even clean my own home any more," cropped up, she learned to rephrase the statement. "Even though there are some things I'm not able to do any more, there are many things I still can do." As she practiced this skill, Debbie's sense of self-worth gradually returned and she began to feel some control over her life again.

Reactions to her illness – shock, denial, frustration, anger – were explored. Debbie was pleased to discover that this was a normal, and necessary, process of adaptation.

Debbie also began to re-evaluate her priorities. She discovered that she had been preoccupied with the accumulation of material goods. She came to realize that this mattered little when placed against the importance of family and friends.

Marital Intervention

Debbie and Mike had enjoyed a happy first few years of marriage, but since the onset of the arthritis both had felt increasingly distant from each other. Since Debbie was tired so much of the time, she and Mike spent much less time going out together, or even just talking. From Mike's perspective, Debbie seemed to have lost interest in him. Although she complained of pain, she looked well to him. The household tasks were no longer being done and Mike even caught himself wondering if she was getting lazy. He was also concerned about Debbie's reduced interest in sex, and when they did make love thoughts that he might be hurting her kept intruding. Debbie, on the other hand, began to feel that Mike wasn't being supportive. She was angry that he didn't help more around the house, and suspected he was worried about the financial consequences if she had to take a leave of absence from her job.

Debbie was relieved that Mike agreed to join us for a series of meetings. It didn't take long for both to realize that they had been experiencing their own emotional reactions to the arthritis, and that the first effect of this was that they were talking less and less to each other.

They began to make adjustments. Mike began to do the grocery shopping and some of the household tasks. They very tentatively learned to clearly express their feelings to each other. They learned to talk openly about their sexual relationship and how each of their needs might be met.

Mike also – and for the first time – went to Debbie's appointment with her rheumatologist, in an attempt to gain a better understanding of her arthritis.

Financial and Vocational Intervention
Debbie and Mike were worried that Debbie might not be able to continue working. They had just purchased a home and were concerned about meeting the mortgage payments on one salary. Resources such as short-term and long-term disability pensions, and vocational rehabilitation, were discussed as potential options. Fortunately for Debbie, she was able to continue teaching. She did make a few changes in her life. She obtained a special "disabled person" parking permit, began to use a chair much more in the classroom, and hired someone to clean the house once a week.

I was pleased with the courage that Debbie and Mike demonstrated in coming to talk to me. I was also pleased that the result appeared to be good – a couple with revised and realistic priorities, with new strategies to cope with chronic illness, and with a relationship now based on honesty and openness. My guess is that they are now closer to each other than ever before.

Group Intervention
To consolidate gains Debbie made in the individual and

marital work, she was referred to a psychosocial group, in order to allow her to interact with others who have arthritis and who were coping with similar challenges.

The group consisted of eight sessions, and was professionally led. In exploring topics of common concern, Debbie found great relief in realizing she was not the only one who was experiencing difficulty in coping with credibility issues, loss of self-esteem and role changes, strong emotional reactions to the diagnosis, changes in her relationships and moodiness due to living with chronic pain. Following the group sessions, Debbie felt a renewed sense of motivation to meet the challenges of living with arthritis.

The Physiotherapist Comments:
When Debbie was first seen, her morning stiffness didn't clear for two hours and she was fatigued all day long. Her hand grip strength was only a third of normal – not surprising in view of the fact that most of her finger joints, along with her left wrist, were swollen, and she was unable even to come close to making a tight fist. In addition to these joints, her shoulders and her foot MTP joints were painful with movement. Her shoulder movement was limited by about 20 percent. Her left knee had a small amount of swelling, but a great deal of pain when she went up and down the stairs at school. In all, she had a total of 20 inflamed joints. She also had decreased strength in her thigh muscles. Neck pain, possibly related to poor posture at work, was an additional problem.

One part of Debbie's job was teaching physical education twice a week. She had always been proud of her physical fitness, but in the past year, due to her pain, stiffness and fatigue, her level of general activity was greatly reduced. It was evident she needed a generalized graded exercise program to regain lost ground.

The problem of pain was partially addressed with the application of ice to all inflamed joints. Debbie purchased ice packs, including extras to use at work. She was shown how to apply them to painful joints, for 15 minutes each session, as frequently as needed. Initially, her left shoulder and left knee received most of this attention, but she also found that applying the pack directly to the soles of her feet gave relief.

I was concerned about the lack of movement in her left wrist and hands, and showed Debbie a general range-of-motion program which involved all her joints, including her neck. I stressed the importance of working this program into her daily schedule, repeating each exercise five times, twice a day. I told her that she might need to use ice applications before each session – and after, if necessary.

Dressing each morning took considerable time, but this (and the duration of her morning stiffness) was shortened considerably after she began starting the day with a hot shower and a run through her exercises.

For neck strain, Debbie was taught posture correction for sitting, standing and lying. She rehearsed this daily, and worked it into her normal activities to the point where she was correcting her posture a minimum of 25 times a day. The emphasis was on chin retraction and pelvic tilting, sitting and standing. A special pillow (Shape of Sleep) was provided, and a high-back Obus Forme was recommended for back support while sitting. Debbie found it particularly helpful when driving and using the computer.

At this stage, with her arthritis far from being controlled, a delicate balance between activity and rest had to be maintained, and this was underlined. She already was well aware of the benefits of good physical fitness. I felt she would benefit from a pool program, and referred her to one led by an experienced physiotherapist. It emphasized achieving a full range of movement of all joints and aimed at a moderate level of conditioning. Later, she progressed to swimming lengths at a neighborhood pool. As her feet became less painful, she resumed her daily half-hour walks in proper footwear. I also told her about a local tai chi program that could improve her overall fitness.

As important as this was, Debbie needed a lot of information and a lot of reassurance. She had been given prescriptions for methotrexate, low-dose prednisone and naproxen. What she had read about the first two quite frankly frightened her, and she had put off getting the prescriptions filled. This isn't uncommon. I gave her pamphlets on them, and discussed with her their benefits and side effects. The importance of regular blood checks, particularly with methotrexate, was stressed. Our information package on RA was also discussed with Debbie.

Two months later, after a total of six treatment sessions, Debbie was discharged from the active physiotherapy case load. I told her that the Arthritis Society would be available if there was a need in the future. She was doing extremely well. Morning stiffness was only 20 minutes, fatigue was delayed until after three p.m., and she no longer needed ice on a daily basis. Knees and feet were much better, and though a number of knuckles were still puffy she had regained 95 percent of her ability to make a fist. She was on a regular home program of resisted isometric exercise for her shoulders and right knee and was beginning to work on her left knee. Neck pain had settled down and she was able to sit at the computer for extended periods without problems. She was still involved in the pool program, once a week, and was swimming on her own at the Y each weekend. Most important of all, she knew much more about her disease and the techniques required for a successful self-management program.

The Occupational Therapist Comments:

My role included vocational intervention, modification of activities of daily living and, to a limited extent, marital intervention.

Vocational Intervention

Debbie and I identified a number of problem areas at work.

Her classroom was on the second floor of the school. Knee and foot pain and fatigue made negotiating stairs painful and difficult. In her classroom, she was experiencing problems raising her arm high enough to write on the blackboard, and gripping the chalk was a challenge. Her desk chair was hard, supported her back poorly, and was without arm rests. Every time she wanted to sit, she had to pull it out from the desk. Writing in her teachers' daily journal was difficult, as was pressing hard enough to make triplicate copies of report cards.

I met the principal of the school and, eventually, his superior at the board. It took some time to implement change but changes were made. These had a marked effect on Debbie's life.

Her classroom was relocated to the main floor, close to the staff room and washroom. The parking spot closest to her class was designated for her exclusive use. She switched to an overhead projector, reducing blackboard use, and when she did use the board she used only the bottom half and gripped the chalk with a special holder. She was given a higher chair to use while writing on overhead transparencies. Her new desk chair had appropriate back support, arm rests and could be adjusted for height. The computer setup was changed to reduce strain on her neck, shoulders and elbows while she was using it.

Physical education classes were rescheduled from ten a.m. to one p.m., and Debbie had a 45-minute break at noon to rest. Two students, assigned in rotation each week, assisted with phys ed equipment setup and storage. Debbie switched from a briefcase to a backpack, reducing the stress on her hands and wrists, and she stopped wearing high heels to work.

Activities of Daily Living

Debbie and I identified quite a few problem areas. She had difficulty applying makeup, doing up small buttons, vacuuming and scrubbing the bathtub.

A large-handled blush applicator was suggested, and she switched from cream blush. A soft eyeliner was recommended. She discovered that a button hook was very helpful in fastening small buttons, particularly when morning stiffness added to her difficulties with dressing. An upright, lightweight vacuum replaced her heavy and awkward canister-style machine. She was encouraged to sit whenever possible when working in the kitchen. She and Mike are considering switching to lever-style handles on the kitchen and bathroom taps.

More than these details, the principles of energy conservation were reinforced – setting priorities, planning, pacing, using appropriate body mechanics and reorganizing her working spaces.

Specific attention was paid to her hands and feet. Splints were made to support her wrists and reduce pain when they are being heavily stressed. Her right index finger had a flexion contracture – it was tight, and was unable to straighten out. This interfered with the use of her hand. I made a splint, designed to stretch the finger out, for her to wear at night. It worked – every two weeks I could see improvement and remolded the splint each time to accommodate the changes.

I taught Debbie to avoid hand activities that might contribute to hand deformities, and suggested she switch to a large-barrel pen, built-up utensils at home and lever-type door knobs and tap handles. I also checked to see that she was doing hand exercises to strengthen muscles and maintain movement.

To replace her high heels, I strongly recommended shoes

with cushioning, a snug heel and adequate toe depth and width, and made sure she knew the name of a store where the staff was knowledgeable. Once she had these, I fitted them with customized insoles (foot orthotics).

Marital Intervention

Debbie and Mike met with me as well. I gave them literature on more comfortable positions during intercourse, but since I knew the social worker had dealt with some of these issues my role was limited. I did, however, discuss my concerns about Debbie's difficulties with heavy household tasks. Mike, who hadn't really thought much about this before these sessions, readily agreed to take on responsibility for these.

Debbie learned about a number of community resources. The Y has activities tailored to people with arthritis. Our arthritis society sponsors a local support group which meets monthly to explore issues of common concern, and as well conducts a program in arthritis self-management. It also has a toll-free telephone line that provides answers to questions about drugs, research, and sources of equipment, and it produces a quarterly publication called *Arthritis News* (see Further Resources).

Surgery

Surgery plays an extremely important role in the treatment of patients with arthritis. However, a surgical consultation is an admission of defeat. Something has happened, with me looking on, that I could not prevent.

These days, however, an admission of defeat doesn't mean a miserable future for the patient. Surgery has made enormous strides in the past 25 years.

When surgical help is sought, it's usually for one of three reasons:

- for relief of severe pain
- for improved function
- to try to prevent something from happening

The first two objectives are most likely to be realized by surgery. Preventive surgery is carried out, however, in certain limited circumstances.

Broadly speaking, arthritis surgery divides into four types – joint replacement, joint fusion, reconstruction, and soft tissue surgery.

Joint Replacement

Joint replacement, pioneered in Great Britain in the late 1960s, has revolutionized orthopedics, bone and joint surgery. It's undoubtedly the greatest single contribution to the welfare of arthritis patients that has been made over the last three decades.

The first problem to be solved was osteoarthritis of the hip. Although prior to the 1960s, artificial joints had been developed, there was no way to keep the parts from slipping. A new "glue" solved the problem. Methyl methacrylate, a bone cement, proved to be a quick-setting, solid attachment for the metal parts, and the boom in joint replacement began.

Since then, the original techniques have been modified many times, because even with the discovery of bone cement there are still problems. The bond between bone and glue and metal does fail occasionally. The metal components themselves may ultimately fracture. If either happens, pain returns and eventually that joint has to be replaced. And second surgeries are never as good as first ones.

So new and stronger metal alloys have been developed. Special surface coatings have been bonded to metal to minimize body tissue reaction to these foreign substances. Components have been fabricated of new, porous materials, designed to encourage new bone to grow into the implanted parts, avoiding the use of glue and, it is hoped, providing an even stronger bond.

Total Hip Replacement (THR)
This surgery was the first, and is still the best. Patients begin to put weight on the joint almost immediately after surgery, and the long-term results are excellent. At least 90 percent of THRs are functioning well after 15 years. With today's models 30 years of use is not an unreasonable expectation, unless the owner is grossly overweight or unusually physically active.

Total Knee Replacement (TKR)
This surgery is almost as good in terms of long-term outcome, although my impression is that a second operation, if necessary, is not as frequently or as completely successful as second THR surgery.

The only other major joints commonly replaced are shoulders and elbows.

Shoulder Replacement
This is usually very successful for pain relief. As long as the ligaments and tendons around the shoulder (the "rotator cuff") have not been severely damaged by the disease process, functional recovery is also quite good. Unfortunately, in rheumatoid arthritis the rotator cuff is frequently damaged and so pain relief, but usually not completely restored function, is the major goal of surgery.

Elbow Replacement
This is done less frequently, and still has a long way to go. Movements of the elbow joint are complex. Unlike the hip

and shoulder, the elbow is not protected by a thick covering of muscle. The older, "hinge" type of elbow replacement was not very satisfactory and I only recommended it for patients with disabling pain. It didn't move like a real elbow, especially in twisting movements. But recently a three-piece elbow joint, looking very much like the three bones that come together at the elbow, has been introduced. I've had a few patients who were delighted with the results – not just with the absence of pain, but with the improvement in function. I hope they continue to be just as happy as time and use test the limits of the hardware.

Deciding on Surgery

When should joint replacement surgery be considered? That's a question that only the patient can answer. It really boils down to "when pain or impaired function is at the point where daily life is becoming very difficult." For two people with similar X-rays, that point might be quite different.

Surgery can be put off too long – particularly if the process has led to major bone loss or significant joint contracture (where the muscles and tendons around the joint became scarred and tight), or if a lot of muscle has been lost through lack of use. If an individual is off his or her feet for three months or more because of knee or hip arthritis, joint replacement surgery usually fails to correct the problem.

An orthopedic consultation should take place before the patient reaches the point where surgery is urgent. That gives the patient and the surgeon a chance to size each other up. It allows time for a clear explanation of the risks and benefits, and for reflection. It also clears the way for a speedy surgical booking when, later, both patient and surgeon agree that the time has come.

Complications of Joint Replacement Surgery

Complications are few. Infection is always a risk, but the figure is now one percent or less. If it occurs, the usual response is to operate again, take out the foreign material, clear the infection with antibiotics and start all over again. It's also recommended that if patients later undergo procedures that may "shower" bacteria into the bloodstream (and thence into the artificial joint), they be given a brief course of antibiotics. Dental surgery and passage of medical instruments into the bladder (cystoscopy) or colon (colonoscopy) are procedures of this type.

Phlebitis (inflammation with obstructing blood clots in the veins of the leg) is a major complication of hip, and to a lesser extent knee, replacement surgery. Because these clots can break loose, pass through the blood vessels to the lungs (pulmonary embolism) and even lead to death, this complication has been the subject of much research. Pulmonary embolism still occurs after approximately 2 percent of hip operations, but the use of blood "thinning" medication, at the time of surgery and after, has made a big difference.

Joint Fusion

The goal of joint fusion, where a bony bridge is surgically constructed across a joint, is to relieve pain and to partially restore function where joint replacement is not possible.

This is most commonly carried out in the wrist and in the ankle region, and is most often done because of severe damage from rheumatoid arthritis. Total joint replacement surgery is not yet sufficiently developed to be used here. Fortunately, post-operative function is surprisingly reasonable, and the relief from pain here makes a huge difference.

Joints are also fused in two uncommon situations:

- where total joint replacement has failed and repeat surgery is technically impossible
- where an artificial joint has been removed because of infection, and, again, repeat surgery would be extremely difficult or impossible

Occasionally, the fusion of a single small joint (the middle joint of the thumb is a good example), converts a useless, unstable thumb into one which can function again in pinching and gripping.

Joint Reconstruction

Technically speaking, total joint replacement fits into this category of surgery. However, what is referred to here is the surgical "cleaning up" (debridement) of damaged bone ends, ligaments and tendons, followed by an attempt to reconstruct a functioning joint with the remaining tissues.

As might be guessed, the success rate of this effort varies. It depends on the disease that caused the damage, how much damage was done and how much work the reconstructed joint has to do.

In rheumatoid arthritis, this type of surgery is commonly done in the forefoot. The joints at the base of the toes, the MTP joints, are the target of prolonged inflammatory damage. As a result, the toes tend to slip upward into a "hammer toe" position, taking with them the protective fat pad over the MTP joint, and leaving the patient to walk painfully on the damaged and inflamed bone ends. Reconstructive surgery involves removing the damaged metatarsal bone ends and the inflamed joint lining (the synovium), pulling the toes back down into alignment and tightening up the ligaments surrounding each joint. Problems with this type of surgery are twofold – a long healing period is necessary before full weight can be put on the foot, and the damage tends to gradually recur under the impact of continuing inflammation and the constant pounding the foot takes with every step.

Reconstructive surgery in the rheumatoid hand is more successful, at least from an appearance perspective. Such deformities as "ulnar drift" of the fingers, and "swan-neck" and "boutonnière" knuckles, can be corrected. Whether or not the use of the hand is improved varies. Prior damage to the joints themselves, and to the small muscles that work the fingers, may be so extensive that the hand looks better but still doesn't work well.

Soft-tissue Surgery

Soft-tissue surgery includes a variety of procedures. These are particularly common in rheumatoid arthritis, where local tissue inflammation can lead to a number of problems:

- in the shoulder, repair of rotator cuff tears (which cause shoulder weakness and pain)
- on the back of the wrist, removal of the thickened, heaped-up, inflamed tendon and joint lining (synovium) when it causes pain and when it threatens to lead to rupture of the tendons that straighten the fingers
- on the inside of the wrist, when pressure on the median nerve causes numbness and tingling in the thumb and first three fingers ("carpal tunnel syndrome"), cutting of the tight ligament that pins the nerve down
- repair of finger tendons that have ruptured, and freeing of tendons that lock or seize up ("trigger fingers"), if local cortisone injections fail

At one time, surgical removal of inflamed rheumatoid tissue from large joints such as the knee was felt to be both effective and necessary. This procedure, called a synovectomy, has been almost entirely abandoned. At best, it bought two years or more of freedom from inflammation in about 50 percent of the joints, but at the cost of a major surgical procedure (including the risk of infection and phlebitis). There are perhaps two other reasons why it's fallen out of favor: general management of RA is much more effective, and results similar to surgical synovectomy can be achieved with injection into the knee of a radioisotope.

Closed synovectomy through an arthroscope – a procedure that involves minimal damage to the muscles and ligaments that cover the joint – is a different matter. It is particularly useful if only one joint is inflamed, and if medicine by mouth or by needle into the joint has failed. A good example is the rare patient with Lyme disease who has persisting pain and swelling in a knee.

Treatment in Pregnancy and Breast-Feeding

Many of my patients get pregnant, have babies and breast-feed. It would be unusual if this were not so, because many forms of arthritis, especially rheumatoid arthritis and lupus, target women in their childbearing years.

These patients have three major concerns:

- what will be the effect of my pregnancy on my arthritis?
- what will be the effect of my arthritis on my pregnancy?
- will drugs affect my baby?

The Effect of Pregnancy on Arthritis

In rheumatoid arthritis it's usually favorable. At least half the women start to feel better within the first three months, and almost three-quarters experience marked improvement sometime during the pregnancy. But a small minority will get worse – about 5 percent – and the remainder will notice no change.

Unfortunately, after delivery, the inflammation returns. In nearly three out of four women this happens within the first two months. Most will have flared up by the end of six months, regardless of whether or not they are breast-feeding. It's distinctly unusual for rheumatoid arthritis to start during pregnancy, whereas it's not at all uncommon for it to begin following the birth of a child. It's almost as if pregnancy "postpones" the disease, and it probably does.

It was the search for the cause of the benefits of pregnancy on RA that led Philip Hench to discover cortisone's effects. And while cortisone clearly has a powerful anti-inflammatory effect, Hench was wrong in believing it was the reason pregnancy improved RA. The answer is much more complex, and is undoubtedly linked to the development of immune tolerance in the mother. This tolerance modifies her immune system to permit the baby, which is in effect a foreign tissue graft much like a transplanted kidney, to survive. In the process, the immune mechanisms that are responsible for so much in RA are suppressed.

Other forms of arthritis don't show such a clear-cut improvement with pregnancy. The few studies that have been done in psoriatic arthritis and ankylosing spondylitis suggest little or no benefit; some women improve, some stay the same and some worsen – in roughly equal numbers.

Pregnancy in systemic lupus erythematosus has been studied extensively, but there does not appear to be any significant effect, for good or ill. Flare-ups of lupus do occur in pregnancy, but they occur at the same rate in similar patients who aren't pregnant. There aren't increased numbers of disease flare-ups or first appearances after delivery – unlike RA.

Carpal tunnel syndrome is common in pregnancy. Fluid

retention and tissue swelling may matter little in most areas, but in the carpal tunnel at the wrist they make a big difference. Pressure on the median nerve appears as wrist and hand pain, numbness and tingling. Since body fluid tends to shift to the arms and hands at night, this is when the symptoms occur. The victim is awakened, and typically gets relief by hanging the arm over the side of the bed and shaking the hand vigorously. Relief comes with delivery, though a carpal tunnel splint worn on the wrist at night can help before then.

The Effect of Arthritis on Pregnancy
Several studies have shown an increased risk of miscarriages (spontaneous abortions), in mothers with rheumatoid arthritis. The expected rate of 10 to 15 percent rises to about 25 percent.

Active systemic lupus erythematosus carries with it a similar increased risk that the pregnancy will be lost. This risk can be reduced somewhat by avoiding pregnancy until the lupus is under good control. But in lupus there are additional factors that may affect pregnancy outcome.

Miscarriages occur not only in the "usual" first trimester (up to 12 weeks), but also in the second trimester. Second-trimester loss is normally quite unusual, and in SLE it appears to be linked to the presence in the blood of the recently discovered "antiphospholipid antibody." This factor is found in some lupus patients, as well as in healthy individuals. In both groups it's tied to delayed miscarriage. It's also linked to an increased risk of blood clot formation in veins (phlebitis) and, occasionally, arteries. There is still debate over what treatment best minimizes the risk to both mother and baby if this blood factor is detected.

An additional and *distinctly uncommon* effect of SLE is on the developing infant heart. A different blood factor, "anti-

Ro antibody," has been linked to complete heart block (but not to an increased miscarriage rate). In this situation, the normal pathways that conduct the heart impulse are injured, causing a permanently slow heartbeat in the baby. This can be detected as early as the 16th week of pregnancy. Fortunately, normal heart action can nowadays be achieved by the implantation of an artificial pacemaker. This seems to be necessary in about half the affected babies.

Anti-Ro antibody also appears to play a role in the development of a lupus-like skin rash in some babies born to mothers carrying that factor. The factor, and the rash, disappear with the passage of time – at least by six months. It should be clearly said, however, that most mothers with anti-Ro antibody will have normal babies.

Arthritis Drugs and the Baby, Before and After Birth

With good reason, most women avoid taking any type of medication during pregnancy. In some cases it's carried to the point where all drugs are stopped as soon as the woman decides to try to get pregnant. On the other hand, many women with arthritis who are on a variety of drugs become pregnant unintentionally. From their experience, and from other situations, a number of conclusions can be reached.

- NSAIDs have not been shown to cause fetal abnormalities, and if they are essential they may be continued in early pregnancy.
- NSAIDs should be avoided in later pregnancy, particularly in the last few months. ASA (aspirin) in particular should be avoided since it has been linked to complications such as prolonged labor, bleeding after delivery and brain hemorrhage in the baby.
- NSAIDs can be taken during breast-feeding if needed.

To minimize the baby's exposure, drugs with a short duration of action, such as ibuprofen, should be used. It has been calculated that if the mother is taking a therapeutic dose of ibuprofen, 400 milligrams four times a day, the baby receives less than 1 milligram. It has also been recommended that the actual medication be taken just as each breast-feeding session begins, assuming that the baby will not feed again for at least four hours.

- "Slow-acting" drugs such as hydroxychloroquine, sulfasalazine, intramuscular gold and even azathioprine have not been shown to affect pregnancy adversely, even though there are theoretical ways they could harm the baby. The situation has to be weighed very carefully, but if the drug is necessary to prevent a flare-up (particularly of lupus) it should be continued. A reduced dose might be tried as one way of cutting the risk. Both sulfasalazine and hydroxychloroquine have been used throughout pregnancy in non-arthritic situations, and seem to have a good record of safety.
- Prednisone may be the safest drug of all, particularly if only low doses are required.
- Cyclophosphamide and methotrexate are *capable of great harm to* the fetus and should never knowingly be taken during pregnancy, although normal pregnancies do occur even with these drugs.

Alternatives to Conventional Medicine

Not too long ago, nobody – neither I nor my patients – talked about this. Now just about all the patients I see ask me about something they've heard about from a neighbor, on television or on the Internet. If I ask, they don't hesitate to tell me what they've tried, or are trying.

I wasn't surprised to read recently that in 1997 it was estimated that $27 billion was spent on "alternative" medicine in the United States (Canada, at one-tenth the population, spends an estimated $3.8 billion Canadian). In one American city, two-thirds of people with appointments to see an arthritis specialist had tried at least one "unconventional" treatment, a quarter had tried three or more and at least half who had tried one were continuing to use it.

The variety of treatments is astounding – chiropractic, copper bracelets, magnets, herbs, electrical stimulators, diet supplements and special diets, minerals and megavitamins, vinegar preparations, acupuncture and spiritual healing. Despite the variety, most of these treatments have one thing in common – they haven't been proved to help the problem for which the person is using them.

As a wise doctor once said, "There is no such thing as alternative medicine – just effective medicine."

It seems clear that many patients choose to pursue two paths at the same time – the "conventional" path I recommend, and the "alternative" path, usually on the grounds that it can't hurt and may help. Use of alternative treatments may also be a marker for significant psychological distress, often depression; this is true of women with breast cancer, and it may be true for people with arthritis as well.

I want to make it clear that I don't criticize a patient who wishes to pursue one of these approaches. I've been around medicine long enough to realize that allopathic medicine (the kind of medicine I practice) has no monopoly on truth – or on untruth.

Dr. Michael Lockshin, a New York rheumatologist and former chair of the Unproven Remedies Committee of the Arthritis Foundation, says people should ask themselves three questions about unproven treatments:

- "Will it hurt me?"
- "Will it cost me a lot of money?"
- "Will it help?"

If I can be sure the answer to the first two is no, I often encourage my patients to find out the answer to the third. I just hope they won't ignore a proven treatment at the same time.

Diet and Arthritis

Should Something Be Dropped from the Diet?
Food allergies are widespread. An extremely conservative estimate is that about 2 percent of the population have an unmistakable food allergy. Egg, wheat, milk, fish and shellfish, nuts, chocolate and citrus fruits are some of the common offenders. Allergic symptoms cover a wide spectrum, from hay fever and asthma symptoms to skin rash, including hives, to gut upset and migraine, to muscle and joint aches and pains.

There have been clear-cut instances where arthritis symptoms in patients diagnosed as having rheumatoid arthritis have come and gone in response to the addition and withdrawal of specific foods given in a "double-blind" fashion. The foods varied by patient, and included corn, wheat, nitrate, shrimp and milk. Most of these patients appeared to be rheumatoid factor (RF) negative. But estimates of the number of RA patients whose symptoms are affected by food are well under 5 percent.

In isolated instances, flare-ups of childhood arthritis and lupus have been linked to specific foods.

A different kind of example is celiac disease, a condition where people are quite intolerant of gluten, a wheat protein. Celiacs often have musculoskeletal symptoms – some quite severe – which improve on a gluten-free diet. I well recall a young woman with intractable pain who, after several years of fruitless investigations and treatment at my hands, saw another doctor who made the correct diagnosis and cured her with diet.

A number of special diets have been studied. Most of these, done in patients with rheumatoid arthritis, started with a period of fasting (often up to a week); then various foods were reintroduced, with or without attempts to avoid specific items. In some instances, a tailored kind of diet was started. The results of these studies have been mixed. Some have shown no benefit. Many others have shown definite benefit, especially during the fasting phase.

One of the most convincing of these demonstrated that a small minority of patients were clearly helped by a diet that eliminated red meat, dairy products, alcohol, preservatives, fruit, herbs and spices. A slightly different study showed that 17 patients put on a long-term vegetarian diet improved and were able to maintain their improvement for at least a year. But nutritionists examining this study have criticized it for two reasons: the numbers were very small, and the diet itself had nutritional deficiencies that could lead to difficulty over the long run.

The conclusion to draw from all of this? There is no blanket prescription. A small number of individuals – probably very few – have food allergies that cause symptoms. In other instances, a vegetarian-type diet may modestly improve the signs and symptoms of inflammation. But medical research continues in this area. I don't think we've heard the last word on dietary manipulation.

Should Something Be Added to the Diet?
Zinc, selenium, copper and vitamins B and C have all been investigated. Addition of these does not affect arthritis.

Eicosopentaneoic acid (EPA) and gammalinolenic acid (GLA) have been shown experimentally to be anti-inflammatory and to blunt immune responses. Fish oils, including cod liver oil, contain EPA. Plant oils, specifically oils from evening primrose and borage, contain GLA. Theoretically, blackcurrant seed oil is even better, because it contains both GLA and a chemical which is converted to EPA.

Studies with these oils have shown that they definitely reduce the "tenderness and pain" index in rheumatoid arthritis, and may affect the extent of the swelling as well. But studies so far have only looked at high doses. It remains to be seen whether lower doses, which would be much easier to take, will be as good.

Seaton is an extract of the New Zealand green-lipped mussel. It appears to have some anti-inflammatory effect in the test-tube and in rats, but well-designed studies haven't turned up any evidence of effectiveness in rheumatoid arthritis or osteoarthritis. And it's expensive.

In the last few years, three dietary supplements – glucosamine (with or without chondroitin), SAM-e and MSM – have become popular. I have already commented on glucosamine – it clearly helps many with the pain of osteoarthritis, but has never been shown to be effective in inflammatory arthritis. SAM-e ("sammy" or S-adenosylmethionine) is an antidepressant and early studies support its claims as a pain reliever. It has also been recommended as an anti-arthritic – but without proof, at least so far. At $1.00 (Canadian) per 100 mg caplet (recommended dosage 4 to 16 a day), it is expensive. Finally, MSM, which is a breakdown product of dimethylsulfoxide (DMSO), is being promoted by a great deal of advertising and word-of-mouth enthusiasm as an arthritis cure. I haven't seen any convincing studies, however, and until I do I'm not going to be recommending it to anyone –

certainly not if I think there is a more effective, proven treatment available.

Herbal Remedies

"All who drink of this remedy are cured, except those who die. Thus it is effective for all but the incurable." – Galen (AD 130–201)

Despite their immense popularity – herbs are, of course, "natural" products and therefore often assumed to be "quite safe" – herbal remedies have not been proved effective in arthritis.

There are many good reasons not to take herbal remedies. Poisoning is one, and it isn't rare. Some cases arise because of contamination and misidentification, but most are probably related to the natural chemistry of the plants themselves. Infants and children appear to be particularly vulnerable.

Another strong reason to be careful with herbal remedies is their potential to interact with conventional drugs for such problems as heart failure, irregular heartbeat patterns, high blood pressure, blood clots, seizures and depression. As a result, conventional drugs may lose their effect – or may have a stronger effect, resulting in a drug overdose.

Some herbal remedies that may be particularly worrisome are gingko, ginseng, feverfew, St. John's wort, shankhapushpi (an Ayurvedic herbal mix), ma huang (Chinese ephedra), devil's claw and plantain. Echinacea, recommended as an immune system stimulant, may be just what someone on immunosuppressive treatment for rheumatoid arthritis or systemic lupus *doesn't* need.

Don't forget that herbs are drugs. Until the active ingredients of an herbal preparation are known, and it is established that the preparation contains a known concentration of them, be careful – especially if you are on conventional drugs. Check with a pharmacist – most should have good information on potential harmful interactions.

In most Western countries, including Canada and the United States, herbal remedies are classified as foods and don't have to pass the more stringent regulations applied to drugs.

Quality control appears to be a big problem. Analysis has shown some preparations to be adulterated with other drugs, and with heavy metals. This is particularly true of products for which there's a huge market – and many unscrupulous individuals wishing to share it.

"Chinese herbal medicines" may contain a variety of herbs and contaminating substances. Deaths due to liver failure, sudden drop in blood pressure and kidney failure have been reported.

Chinese proprietary medicines deserve special mention. These are very popular, and not only in the Far East. An elderly Chinese lady with rheumatoid arthritis is a patient of mine. She has taken Chinese proprietary medicines for some time – she gets them from relatives in Hong Kong. She's delighted with their effect, and won't hear of stopping them. I did persuade her to bring me the package, and printed on the side were the ingredients of each tablet – a cortisone-like drug, two different NSAIDs (one restricted in Canada) and a painkiller. Some of these ingredients were in laughably low doses, others in doses higher than I would use. Similar preparations obtainable in Hong Kong and presumably contaminated (I hope hers isn't) have been linked to mercury, lead, cadmium and arsenic poisoning.

Periodically, I discover that a patient has obtained some arthritis remedy from Mexico. When these have been analyzed, they too invariably contained cortisone-like drugs and an NSAID – a combination with high risk for side effects.

Finally, let me say something positive about herbal remedies. Many have been around a very long time. Tradition does say something about safety and effectiveness. We just need to know more about them. We need to isolate the chemicals unique to each herb and test them carefully, first in the laboratory and then in the clinic.

A good example of this is the Chinese herb known as thunder god vine, a remedy that has been used for years in China to treat rheumatoid arthritis. Its active ingredient – triptolide – has been isolated. It has now been tested in the lab and shown to keep immune cells from turning on the inflammation chain reaction (it may also have anti-cancer actions). The leap from the lab to the pharmacy is a big one, but if tests in humans prove successful we may soon have another weapon to use against such conditions as rheumatoid arthritis and systemic lupus.

Acupuncture

In 1972 – coincident with Richard Nixon's trip to China – the Western world "discovered" acupuncture. The theory of acupuncture attributes illness to an imbalance of body energy forces. Based on an assessment of this imbalance, needles are inserted beneath the skin according to a predetermined pattern. The pattern is dictated by which "meridian" of the body system was out of balance, as well as by the influences – Wind, Cold, Fire, Dampness, Dryness and Summer Heat – that might be affecting this imbalance.

I think I can safely make several statements about acupuncture:

- It has never been shown to *cure* any disease.
- When needle placement is made at traditional Chinese locations, a pain-relieving effect can be detected.

- This pain-relieving effect is superior to the effect (which can also be detected) of needle placement in nearby sites which are not those prescribed by traditional Chinese practice.
- Acupuncture needle stimulation in experimental animals causes release of natural painkillers (endorphins).
- Acupuncture seems to have a definite role in the treatment of both acute and chronic musculoskeletal pain. Studies of longstanding low back pain have been particularly impressive.
- It seems to work best when it's co-ordinated with a variety of other approaches – physiotherapy, fitness and muscle strengthening, behavioral modification.
- There are various schools of acupuncture. None has shown its superiority over any other.

My advice? Acupuncture is worth a try, particularly if you're attempting to deal with longstanding, disabling, non-inflammatory pain. Just don't give up on the other things I also recommend.

Homeopathy

Homeopathy is based on the "Law of Similars." The first principle of homeopathy holds that a condition can be treated by administering a substance which, in full strength, causes symptoms similar to the disease to be treated. An 18th-century German physician, Samuel Hahnemann, popularized this principle after taking a strong dose of cinchona bark – which contains the antimalarial quinine – and experiencing headache, thirst and fever – all symptoms of malaria. With friends, he began experimenting with various herbs and other substances, making careful notes on the symptoms produced. He then moved on to develop the second principle of homeopathy – that if a large dose of a substance causes symptoms of a given disease, then extremely small doses will cure it. The smaller the dose, the stronger the medicine.

The difficulty most conventional doctors have with the theory is that the dilutions are carried to such an extreme that the laws of chemistry make it infinitely unlikely that any given bottle will contain a single molecule of the substance. A standard "30C" strength of saline, for instance, is comparable to one molecule of salt dissolved in a volume of water equivalent to all this planet's waters. But homeopathy rises above the mathematics. It concludes that the alcohol or water of the solution develops a "memory" of the substance to which it has been exposed, and that it's this "memory" that has the desired effect.

So much for the theory. Does homeopathy work? Again we come to controlled studies, and again the data just aren't there. There has been only one acceptable study in rheumatoid arthritis. In contrast to a number of other reports that showed no benefit, it demonstrated a reduction in pain in patients receiving homeopathic treatment. This study has been criticized on the grounds that patients weren't assigned in a random fashion to one group or the other, and so it does not meet strict study criteria.

To be fair, there have been a very few studies that were well designed and showed treatment benefits in flu, hay fever and infant diarrhea. But like any research results, these should be repeated successfully before they are fully accepted. In the United States, the National Institutes of Health now includes an Office of Alternative Medicine. I only hope it will foster the work that needs to be done to lay this and other issues to rest.

In the meantime, while I certainly wouldn't recommend them, homeopathic remedies seem harmless enough – as long as using them doesn't mean postponing treatment that is known to be effective.

Chiropractic

The most common symptom for which people seek alternative medicine is back pain. And the most commonly sought out alternative practitioner is the chiropractor.

In 1990 *The British Medical Journal* reported on two groups of patients with low back pain. One group was treated by chiropractors, one by physiotherapists. At the end of two years, the chiropractic-treated group felt better – but they had been treated more intensively, at a greater cost, over the two years. Nevertheless, this outcome was viewed as a vindication of those who advocated chiropractic.

More recently, *The New England Journal of Medicine* reported a two-year study of similar low-back-pain sufferers. Here, though, there were three groups – a chiropractic group, a physiotherapy group and a group that was given an educational pamphlet on low back pain. The outcome was similar in all three groups – particularly in terms of days off work, reduced activity and return of pain. The booklet group had slightly but not significantly more symptoms, but was definitely less happy (30 percent happy) about the treatment given, compared to the other two groups (75 percent happy).

What do I conclude from all this? Back pain gets better in almost anyone, but the laying on of hands – by a chiropractor or a physiotherapist – makes people happier. That is no mean achievement, and I don't hesitate to recommend one or the other to my patients. But first I make sure that the back pain is not a signal of an underlying condition in which delay or chiropractic manipulation would be harmful.

And All the Rest

Regular newspaper readers will recognize WD-40 oil, DMSO (dimethyl sulfoxide), copper bracelets, bee venom, honey and vinegar, and sitting in abandoned radium mines as all making claims to effectiveness in arthritis. Unfortunately, at this time that's all they are. Claims.

I don't pretend to have all the answers. I recognize that the theory behind a lot of what we have done in arthritis treatment has been faulty, and that quite a lot of what was done not so very long ago was worthless and even harmful.

The best I can do is attempt to evaluate current practice honestly, tell my patients what we do and don't know, and let them decide. If they decide to pursue unconventional medicine, as long as they do it with full knowledge of the uncertainties and the alternatives, I can't criticize their choice.

> *"I didn't say there was nothing better,"* the King
> replied. *"I said there was nothing like it."*
> – *Lewis Carroll*, Through the Looking Glass

Glossary

(Some definitions refer to "skeleton" – see diagram preceding Chapter 1.)

Anemia: A condition in which the number of red blood cells (responsible for carrying oxygen from the lungs to body tissues) is lower than normal. The two most common reasons for anemia are (1) excessive blood loss (such as from a bleeding stomach ulcer) and (2) defective manufacture of new blood cells (which is a common problem in many chronic diseases). Both may contribute to anemia in some forms of arthritis.

Antibody: A protein molecule, made by a specialized white blood cell (the B-lymphocyte). Antibodies are normally custom-made to help protect the body against foreign proteins (known as antigens). The body encounters many antigens every day – viruses, bacteria, drugs are some. In some forms of arthritis, antibodies are formed against normal body proteins and disease symptoms may result from this "autoimmune" reaction. Rheumatoid factor (RF) is an auto-antibody of this type.

Arthralgia: Pain in one or many joints (used when swelling is not observed).

Arthroplasty: Surgery carried out on a joint in an attempt to improve its function. Artificial joint surgery, such as a total knee arthroplasty, fits into this category.

Arthroscopy: A procedure that involves introducing a small diameter flexible fiberoptic cable, through the skin, into a joint. This allows the interior of the joint to be examined. Almost any joint can be examined in this fashion, but the knee is most commonly arthroscoped. Surgery can also be performed at the same time by introducing similarly small instruments into the joint and operating under direct arthroscopic vision.

Bursa: A sac-like structure found over many places on the body where pressure is applied. Many bursae are just beneath the skin (such as the olecranon bursa, covering the tip of the elbow) and others are deeper. A bursa in its normal "collapsed" state is similar to a small deflated balloon that contains a few drops of fluid. It allows the overlying tissues to roll over the bony bump without tearing. If the bursa is injured or inflamed, it may swell and become tense and painful – a condition called bursitis.

Cartilage: The tough whitish covering of the ends of bones where they come together in a joint. Cartilage permits smooth, low friction movement. When it deteriorates, the process known as osteoarthritis develops.

Claudication: Leg pain coming on when the blood supply can't provide the necessary oxygen to the exercising muscles. It is relieved by resting the muscles or by doing something (usually surgical) to improve the circulation. One form of back disease (spinal stenosis) can cause pain very similar to vascular claudication.

Collagen: The most abundant protein in the body, usually formed in thick tough strands, that provides strength and shape to many body structures, including cartilage, skin, and heart valve tissues.

Connective tissue disease: A term that is about as meaningless as "arthritis." Connective tissue consists of the cells, fibers (including collagen), and semi-liquid "glue" that hold tissues together. At one point about 30 years ago, it was proposed that the common denominator in a wide variety of conditions (including rheumatoid arthritis, lupus erythematosus, polymyositis and scleroderma) was a defect in connective tissue. It's still used as a useful shorthand for referring to such diseases, but shouldn't be taken to imply that connective tissue is anything more than an innocent bystander.

COX: An enzyme, cyclooxygenase, that initiates the production of inflammatory chemicals. COX is the target for the NSAID group of drugs.

CT (or CAT) scan: The acronym stands for "computerized axial tomography." This is a process whereby the technology of X-ray and that of the computer are combined, producing an image of body tissues previously unavailable. We use it in rheumatology to look at bone and, in particular, the spine.

Dactylitis: Dactyls are fingers and toes. Inflammation may cause individual toes or fingers to become diffusely swollen and red – hence "dactylitis."

DIP joints: The joints at the ends of the fingers. DIP=distal interphalangeal (see skeleton).

Disc (or disk): The puck-shaped cushion between individual vertebrae, or bones of the spine. Its outer layers consist of thick strands of tightly wound collagen, like the outer layers of a golf ball, and – like a golf ball – its center is a semiliquid gel. This permits the disc to act as a "shock-absorber." With age, the center of the disc tends to dry up, causing a shrinkage in disc height.

Edema: The accumulation of increased, and abnormal, amounts of water in body tissues. The swelling of ankles and feet during pregnancy is due to edema.

Enthesis: The point where ligaments and tendons attach to bone. Inflammation at this point is called an "enthesitis." A "tennis elbow" and a "heel spur" are examples of enthesitis.

Epicondyles: The bony "knobs" on the inside and the outside of the elbow joint (where the forearm muscles are attached).

Fascia: A tough sheet of tissue, usually just under the skin, which covers and protects underlying structures. One such layer covers the outside of the thigh from pelvis to knee; another covers the sole of the foot from the base of the toes to the heel. Fasciitis refers to inflammation of this tissue.

Intra-articular: Literally, "within the joint."

Lumbar/lumbosacral: Refers to the lower five vertebrae of the spine (the lumbar spine). Lumbosacral extends the reference to include the sacrum, the curved segment at the base of the spine (see skeleton).

MCP joints: The joints at the base of the fingers that form the near row of knuckles. MCP = metacarpophalangeal (see skeleton).

Microsurgery: Surgery carried out with the help of a magnifying apparatus. In bone and joint surgery, microsurgical disc surgery is sometimes carried out in an attempt to be less injurious to the surrounding tissues.

Monarticular: Literally, involving a single joint.

MTP joints: The joints at the base of the toes that form the "ball" of the foot. MTP = metatarsophalangeal (see skeleton).

Musculoskeletal: Refers to muscles, bones and joints.

NSAID: An acronym for nonsteroidal anti-inflammatory drugs, pronounced "ensaid." Includes ASA (aspirin) and a host of others such as ibuprofen, indomethacin and naproxen. Painkillers such as acetaminophen are not NSAIDs.

Occupational therapy: One of the health professions involved in helping patients with arthritis adapt to their disease and their environment (see section on Treatment).

Orthopedic: An adjective that refers to the correct positioning of the skeleton. Orthopedic surgery is that branch of surgery aiming at correcting skeletal disorders, including fractures and the damage done by arthritis.

Orthotic: A device, such as a splint or insole, designed to support a part of the skeleton in its normal position or posture.

Ostcoporosis: A condition where the solidity of bone is greatly reduced by an excess of normal bone breakdown over bone repair (see section on Corticosteroids).

Osteotomy: A surgical incision into bone designed to change its alignment.

Phlebitis: Inflammation of a vein. When this is accompanied by the development of a blood clot (thrombosis) in the inflamed segment of vein, as it often is, the term "thrombophlebitis" is used.

Physiotherapy: A method of treatment designed to restore function in the musculoskeletal system. Strong emphasis is placed on exercise.

PIP joints: Proximal interphalangeal (PIP) joints form the "middle" knuckles halfway down the fingers and toes.

Plantar: Refers to the bottom of the foot. In the hand, the equivalent term is "palmar."

Polyarthritis: Literally, "many(poly-) joints(arthr-) inflamed(-itis)." This is usually qualified by an adjective such as "seronegative" (that is, the rheumatoid factor test is negative) or "symmetrical" (that is, both right and left sides of the body are similarly affected).

Prosthesis: A man-made replacement for a normal body part (in orthopedic surgery, this may mean anything from an artificial joint to an artificial leg).

Rheumatoid factor: An antibody found in the blood in about 5 percent of the normal population, but found in the blood of 60 percent or more of those who have rheumatoid arthritis (and sometimes other forms of arthritis as well).

Rheumatologist: A medical doctor who specializes in the prevention, diagnosis and non-surgical treatment of the many forms of arthritis.

Seropositive: Medical jargon that implies that the blood test for a condition was positive (a patient can be "seropositive" for HIV, or mononucleosis, or syphilis – but in patients with arthritis it usually is taken to mean that the blood test for rheumatoid factor is positive).

Spondylarthritis: The variety of inflammatory arthritis that affects the spine and, often, the joints of the arms and legs. Ankylosing spondylitis and psoriatic arthritis are examples.

Synovium: The membrane lining the joint. It makes the lubricating fluid of the joint, and in inflammatory arthritis it becomes very inflamed and thickened and plays an important role in the joint damage that occurs.

Tophus (plural form, tophi): A mass of crystals of sodium urate, collected together in a "lump" under the skin, that may be detected in individuals with gout.

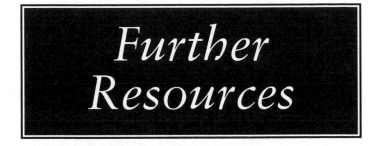

Further Resources

Organizations

The offices listed below are national; for regional branches, check your telephone directory.

Canada

Arthritis Society of Canada
393 University Ave.
Suite 1700
Toronto, ON M9G 1E6
1-800-321-1433
(416) 979-3760
Fax: (416) 979-8366
www.arthritis.ca

Separate associations for fibromyalgia, juvenile arthritis, lupus, scleroderma and spondylitis operate under the auspices of the Arthritis Society.

U.S.

The American Juvenile Arthritis Organization operates under the auspices of the Arthritis Foundation.

The Arthritis Foundation
PO Box 7669
Atlanta, GA 30357-0669
1-800-283-7800 (Automated)
(404) 872-7100
www.arthritis.org

American Lyme Disease Foundation
293 Route 100
Somers, NY 10589
1-800-876-LYME (Automated)
(914) 277-6970
www.aldf.com

Fibromyalgia Network
PO Box 31750
Tucson, AZ 85751-1750
1-800-853-2929
(520) 290-5508
www.fmnet.news

Lupus Foundation of America
1300 Piccard Dr., Suite 200
Rockville, MD 20850-4303
(301) 670-9292
www.lupus.org

National Psoriasis Foundation
6600 SW 92nd Ave., Suite 300
Portland, OR 97223-7195
1-800-723-9166 (Automated)
(503) 244-7404
www.psoriasis.org

Scleroderma Foundation
89 Newbury St., Suite 201
Danvers, MA 01923
1-800-722-4673
(978) 750-4499
www.scleroderma.org

Sjögren's Syndrome
    Foundation Inc.
366 North Broadway
Jericho, NY 11753
1-800-475-6473
(Automated; U.S. only)
(516) 933-6365
www.sjogrens.com

Spondylitis Association
    of America
1-800-777-8189 (U.S. only)
www.spondylitis.org

Books

Aladjem, Henrietta. *The Challenges of Lupus: Insights and Hope.* New York, NY: Avery, 1999.

———. *Understanding Lupus.* New York, NY: Charles Scribner's Sons, 1985.

Hall, Hamilton. *The Back Doctor.* Toronto, ON: Seal, 1982.

Horstman, Judith. *The Arthritis Foundation's Guide to Alternative Therapies.* Marietta, GA: Longstreet Press, 1999.

Hunder, Gene (ed.). *Mayo Clinic on Arthritis.* New York, NY: Kensington, 1999.

Kelly, Julie. *Taking Charge of Fibromyalgia.* Fibromyalgia Educational Systems, 1998.

Lorig, Kate, and James N. Fries. *The Arthritis Helpbook* (4th edition). Reading, MA: Perseus, 1995.

Shlotzhauer, Tammi, and James McGuire (ed.). *Living with Rheumatoid Arthritis* (Johns Hopkins Health Book). Baltimore, MD: Johns Hopkins, 1995.

Wallace, Daniel. *The Lupus Book: A Guide for Patients and Their Families.* New York, NY: Oxford, 1996.

Wallace, Daniel, and Janice Wallace. *Making Sense of Fibromyalgia.* New York, NY: Oxford, 1999.

Magazines

Arthritis News (quarterly) Available through the Canadian Arthritis Society (address above).

Arthritis Today (every two months) Available through the American Arthritis Foundation (address above).

Websites

A great deal of misinformation is out there on the Web. The following sites contain arthritis-related information that I find reliable. See also Organizations, above.

www.altmedicine.com	Alternative Health News Online
www.altmednet.com	Alternative Medicine Alert
www.fda.gov/fdac	U.S. Food and Drug Administration
www.nih.gov/niams	National Institute of Arthritis and Musculoskeletal and Skin Diseases (National Institutes of Health)
www.quackwatch.com	Quackery Related Topics

Index

Page numbers in italic indicate that the cited information is on that page only in a figure or box.